I0758659

The content of this book is for informational purposes only. Never consume any wild plants unless you are completely certain they are safe to eat. It's vital to verify information gathered online with input from an expert, a foraging group, or multiple reliable resources. Enjoy the activity, but act with caution. Accurate identification is your responsibility and could very well determine your safety.

Do not eat wild plants unless you are skilled in recognizing and safely preparing them. Do not forage or gather wild edible plants in protected or restricted zones without a permit. The author excludes all liability for any harm, injury, or cost inflicted, directly or indirectly, from the use, consumption, or contact with plants mentioned in "Foraging Horta."

The author offers no assurances regarding the safety of any food or drink made using the plants in this publication. The author is not liable for any health issues or losses arising from using or consuming products made by the buyer with the plants described in this book, including any recipes or suggested preparations.

The book is also not intended to diagnose, treat, cure, or prevent any condition or disease. You understand that this book is not intended as a substitute for consultation with a licensed practitioner. Please consult with your own physician or healthcare specialist regarding the suggestions and recommendations made in this book.

The use of this book implies your acceptance of this disclaimer.

First edition: November 2024

ISBN: 9798751153014 {KDP}

CONTENTS

Eat Your Greens, the Greek Way   6

A Little History   8

How to Prepare Horta at Home   12

56 Types of Horta You'll Find in Crete   15

Agoglossos (Anchusa azurea)   16

Agriagginara (Cynara cornigera)   17

Ágrio spanáki (Rhagadiolus edulis)   18

Agriovrouva (Sisymbrium officinale)   20

Agriolàchano (Brassica cretica subsp. aegaea)   21

Agrios Maïntanós (Scaligeria napiformis—syn. Scaligeria cretica)   22

Agriópraso (Allium ampeloprasum)   23

Agriosélino (Apium nodiflorum)   24

Akournópodas (Oenanthe pimpinelloides)   25

Amáranto (Limonium sinuatum)   26

Ascordulakas (Muscari comosum)   28

Askordoúlakas áspros (Ornithogalum narbonense)   29

Ascolympros (Scolymus hispanicus)   30

Chátzikas (Scandix pecten veneris L.)   31

Chinopódio (Chenopodiastrum murale)   33

Choiromourída (Helminthotheca echioides)   34

Galatsída (Reichardia picroides)   35

Gérontas (Urospermum picroides)   36

Glystrída (Portulaca oleracea)   37

Kápari (Capparis spinosa)   39

Kardamo (Capsella bursa pastoris)   40

Kavkalíthra (Tordylium apulum)   41

Klouvída (Chenopodium album)   42

Kokkinogoúli (Crepis vesicaria)   43

Korakoúli (Scabiosa atropurpurea)   44

Koutsounáda (Papaver rhoeas)   45

Krítamos (Crithmum maritimum)   46

Lagoudóchorto (Prasium majus)   47

Lápatho (Rumex acetosa)   48

Leivadítis (Pimpinella peregrina)   49

Mantilída (Glebionis coronaria)   50

Máratho (Foeniculum vulgare)   51

Melissóchorto (Melissa officinalis)   52

Molócha (Malva sylvestris)   53

Pentaneuro (Plantago major)   54

Perdikoúli (Anagallis arvensis)   55

Petromároulo (Lactuca serriola)   56

Petrofiliá (Petromarula pinnata)   57

Pigounítis (Tragopogon sinuatus)   58

Pikróvrouva (Hirschfeldia incana)   59

Pikrorádiko (Taraxacum officinale)   60

Pirounáki (Erodium cicutarium)   61

Radíki (Cichorium intybus)   62

Rapanída (Raphanus raphanistrum)   63

Sparángi (Asparagus aphyllus)   65

Stamnankáthi (Cichorium spinosum)   66

Starída (Hedypnois cretica)   67

Stafylinakas (Daucus carota)   68

Striftoúli (Scorpiurus muricatus)   69

Stroufoúli (Silene vulgaris)   70

Stýfnos (Solanum nigrum)   72

Tsichlántero (Stellaria cupaniana)   73

Tsouknída (Urtica pilulifera)   74

Tsóchos (Sonchus oleraceus)   76

Xynída (Oxalis pes-caprae)   77

Vlita (Amaranthus retroflexus)   78

REFERENCES   84

Eat Your Greens, the Greek Way

In Greece, eating horta is a way of life. Though their name may literally translate to "weeds," these wild edibles are considered far from that—they're valuable delicacies.

Horta is a generic name given to a vast variety of wild greens; some 300 edible species grow here, according to Greek and Mediterranean cuisine expert Diane Kochilas. Each season has its own. Spring brings the greatest abundance of young greens, among them dandelion, grass lily, borage, and wild garlic and leeks. In the summer, you will find plenty of amaranth leaves and purslane; while fall and winter are the seasons for reichardia and wild chicories. You'll never go hungry feeding off the land.

Passing down ages-old knowledge, grandmothers teach their grandchildren how to forage for horta in the wild, because they know the best grow along mountain slopes and hillsides, in olive groves, and on fertile plateaus. Armed with pocket knives and baskets or tote bags, they hunt for just the right patch of young leaves, teaching the little ones how to discern the edible from the inedible. They cut the greens just above the soil, leaving the roots to allow the plant to regrow, then carry their harvest back home for a feast.

Greeks have been eating horta since ancient times. Rich in vitamins, minerals, and myriad other nutritional benefits, these gifts of the land provided crucial sustenance during the lean, hard years of war. Now, even supermarkets sell them, alongside cultivated varieties like chard and mustard greens. Still, cultivated horta doesn't taste like "the real thing"—the wild greens that take their nutrients naturally from the land, rain, wind, and sunshine, without human intervention. Horta are a staple in Greek households and on taverna menus, with the varieties changing by the season.

Whenever I dine out with friends here in Crete, they'll invariably order a plate—among many others to share. The most typical preparation is also the simplest, the same regardless of the variety: boiled until tender or still slightly crunchy, then chilled in icy water, drained, and seasoned with salt, good olive oil, and fresh lemon juice. Slightly bitter, with earthy notes, they're served as is, or with a combo of boiled zucchini, potatoes, and half a lemon. It's unpretentious, honest food, light and nourishing.

You can use most horta leaves in about any recipe that calls for spinach, chard, kale, etc.

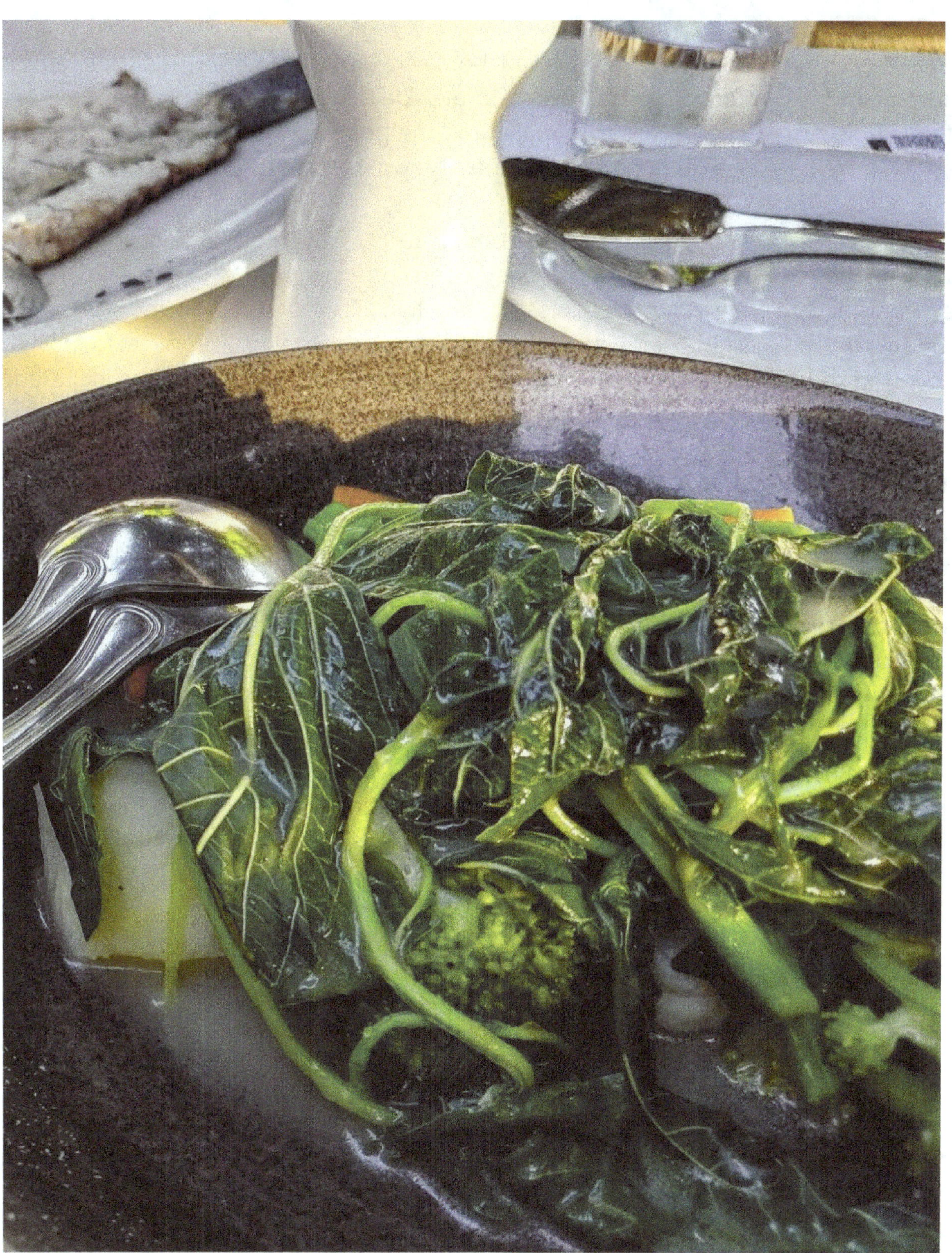

Horta with boiled vegetables in a Cretan restaurant.

A Little History

Minoan frescoes illustrate the deep bond between the Cretans and their surroundings, featuring vivid depictions of plants integral to their daily life and spiritual rituals. In contrast to the Middle Ages, when grasses primarily fed the poor and farmers, Cretan diets stood apart. Wild plants were vital during tough times like wars, occupations, and poor harvests.

The diverse Cretan vegetation ensured the people rarely faced hunger. Local culinary habits influenced the choice of veggies and shaped cooking techniques. Wild greens, full of plant fibers, aid digestion and optimize digestive function. They are rich in minerals, such as calcium, iron, potassium, sodium, magnesium, and manganese. They also provide B vitamins, vitamin C, and pro-vitamin A. Global diets, including Greece's, have included wild greens for centuries. Eaten both fresh and cooked, these plants have been part of culinary traditions since antiquity. With its rich natural environment, Crete has long enabled its residents to incorporate wild edibles into their meals.

The region's greenery consistently graced local tables. Remarkably, all the greens documented by Byzantine writers remain edible in Crete today. During Venetian rule, Cretans extensively used native plants for medicinal purposes. The longstanding tradition of olive oil production and its export from Crete, originating in the Minoan times and continuing today, plays a crucial role in the high consumption of greens.

Every Cretan, whether residing in rural or urban areas, even outside Crete, typically has their own olive oil supply. When cooking greens, ample oil is needed for flavor. Thus, consumption is less in regions abundant with greens but lacking olive oil.

Carotenes, Omega-3s, and other phytochemicals from secondary plant metabolism, such as phenols and terpenes, are essential to human health. These substances have hormonal, enzymatic, antioxidant, antibacterial, antimicrobial, and anticancer effects. They do not cause fat-related stress and are low in carbohydrates and protein, supplementing rather than forming the diet's basis.

Most wild greens have healing properties that can boost well-being and aid recovery. Compared to cultivated greens, wild plants might be free from chemical contaminants like pesticides and fertilizers if sourced from uncontaminated areas.

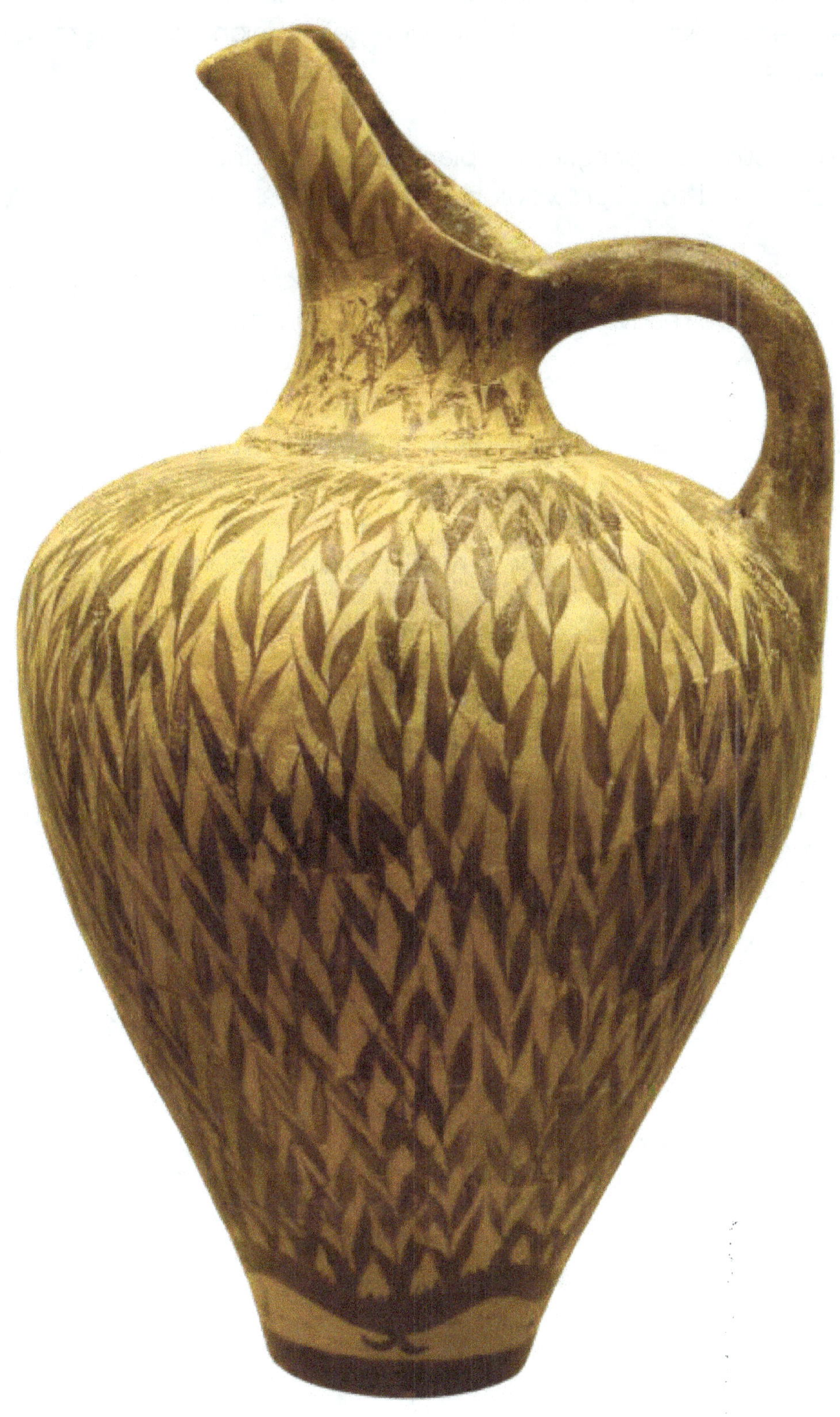

Late Minoan New-Palace period (1450 BCE) clay jug with distinctive leaf pattern, from Phaistos. (Heraklion Archaeological Museum, Crete)

Got weeds in your yard? Many of the plants we often call weeds are actually edible and packed with nutrients. Learning about these wild greens might even make pulling weeds a more enjoyable task.

From the first dandelions of spring, edible plants are all around. Stinging nettles pop up near berry bushes, and wood sorrel grows along garden edges.

You can fill bowls with wild greens for salads and cooking long before planted crops, like lettuce or amaranth, are ready. These edible treasures include leafy greens, roots, flowers, berries, and stems.

The variety of wild edibles is impressive. Garlic mustard has a flavor reminiscent of mustard greens with a hint of garlic. Other options include plantain, curly dock, cress, and chicory, all growing abundantly nearby. Even violets and violas, with their leaves and tiny blooms, can be eaten, often adding color and flavor to meals. Foraging has grown in popularity, exciting both rural and urban dwellers.

Why eat wild plants? There are plenty of benefits to consider.

Rich in nutrients: Wild greens often have more antioxidants, vitamins C and E, and beta-carotene than horta. They thrive in challenging environments, developing higher levels of minerals compared to many cultivated crops.

Good for health: A diverse diet is essential. Grocery stores provide only a small fraction of edible plants. Eating a variety of wild foods helps you incorporate more vitamins and minerals into your meals. It may take some experimenting to find recipes you enjoy, but the rewards are worth it.

Disease-fighting properties: Wild plants produce natural compounds to protect themselves from threats like UV radiation, bacteria, and fungi. These same compounds can benefit humans by acting as antioxidants, anti-inflammatories, or even mild antibiotics.

Connecting to nature: Foraging for wild food is deeply fulfilling. It strengthens our bond with nature and links us to our hunter-gatherer ancestors.

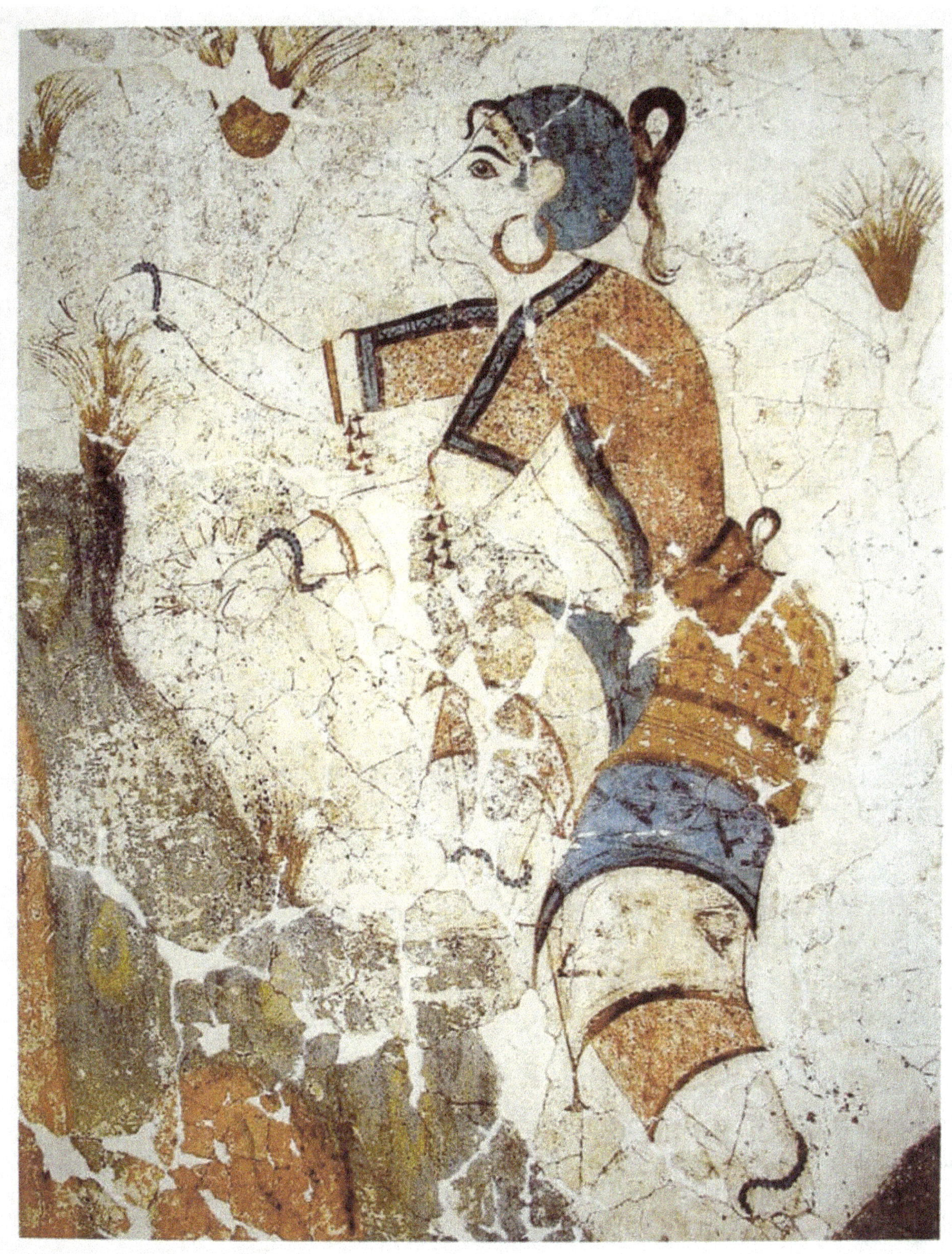

Minoan girl gathering Crocus. Fresco from Akrotiri (Xeste 3, Room 3, 1st floor), 17th century BC. Now in the Prehistoric Museum of Thira, Fira, Santorini.

How to Prepare Horta at Home

There are no set-in-stone recipes for horta, nor rules for the varieties you can use. Follow your heart—and whatever seasonal leafy greens are available near you, whether foraged yourself or purchased from your local farmers market.

Even here in Heraklion, on Crete, I don't forage for my own greens. I go to mom-and-pop mini markets whose owners are more than happy to recommend their freshly foraged finds, and repeat over and over how to cook them: wash thoroughly, discarding the water several times, then boil, drain, let it cool. Season with salt, drizzle with a generous amount of olive oil and freshly squeezed lemon juice, and serve.

The most challenging part of the process is the cleaning. It may take up to half an hour to pick out the dead leaves, grass, twigs, and dirt from the horta. As Nefteria, the owner of a mini-market across the road, always tells me,

"Wash, wash, wash!" It's sweet how she repeats it every time, although I know it; it feels maternal.

As simple as the preparation is, there are some tricks to making horta enjoyable, to tame their bitter taste. At the family-owned taverna To Mourelo tou Ladomenou in Galatas, a small inland village in Heraklion, chef Grigoris Koudounas always has seasonal horta on the menu. It is never bitter.

"Change the water a couple of times when you boil them," he told me.

"You must cool the horta in ice-cold water every time you change the boiling water, to maintain the vibrant green of the plants." I know his trick now—I'll cook better.

There's also more to horta than boiling: The greens can instead be sautéed in olive oil, as in horta tsigarista, or baked into a phyllo-crusted pie, called hortopita. Still, I prefer boiled horta, the easiest and simplest way to prepare them. If you are fully committed to the horta lifestyle, and the traditional resourceful, no-waste spirit it embodies, don't discard the broth from the last boil. I dare you to drink it—it's like an earthy-bitter, medicinal, herbal tea.

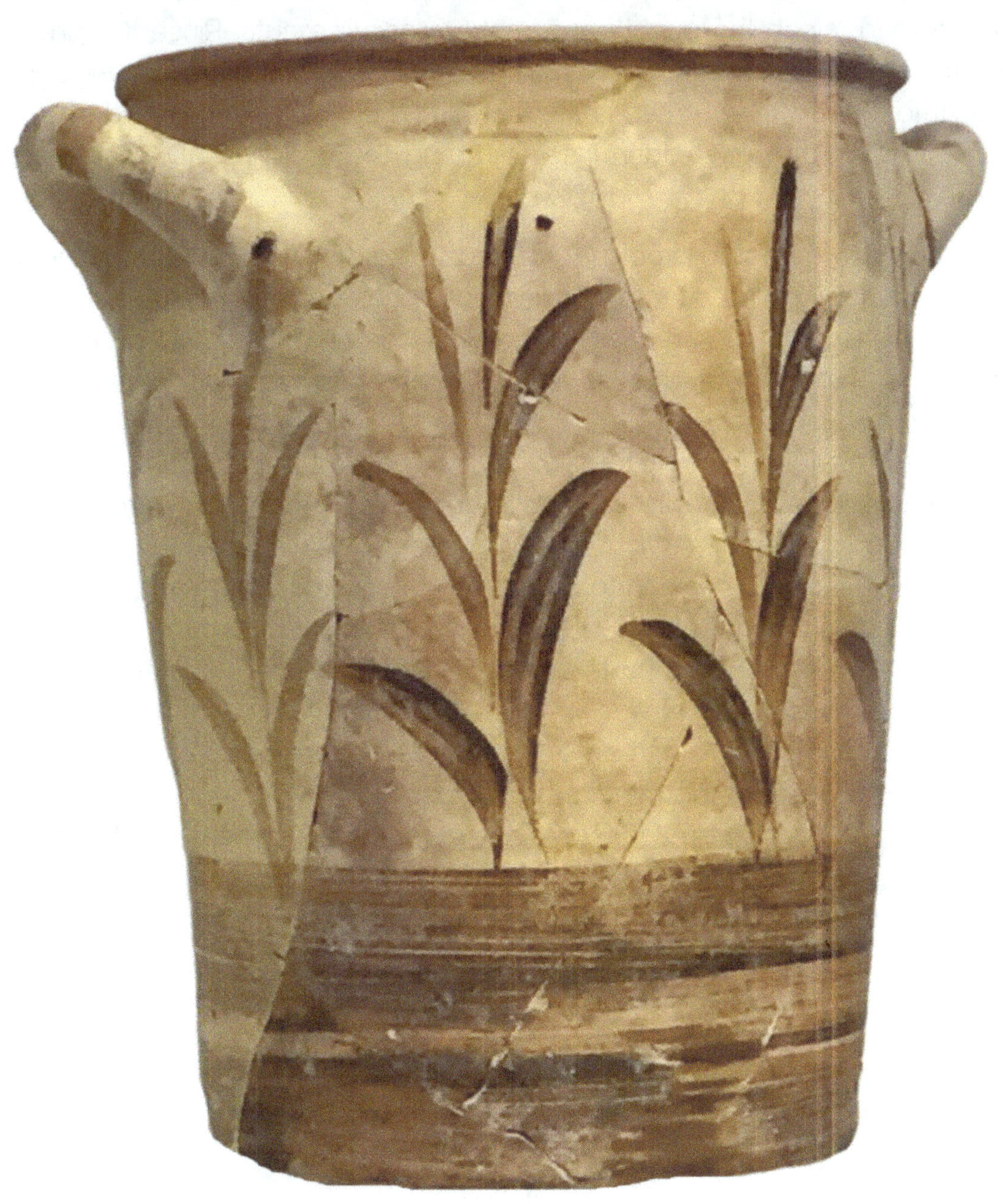

Late Minoan New-Palace period (1450 BCE) clay jug with distinctive leaf pattern, from Phaistos. (Heraklion Archaeological Museum, Crete)

- **Selecting Horta:** Select bright green horta with firm stalks. Avoid those with soft stalks, wilted leaves, or yellow/black spots. These indicate they are not fresh. The horta in supermarkets is usually cultivated (not wild) and clean. Before cooking, you will still need to clean it and look for wilted or darkened stems and leaves.

- **Cleaning:** Begin by meticulously cleaning the wild greens, paying special attention to those with short leaves and roots. Never remove the root stem, as it holds the most flavor. Instead, clean thoroughly and make crosswise cuts. Rinse the greens well in water to remove soil and impurities. Fill a large basin with water, plunge the greens, and agitate them with your hands. Repeat until the water is clear. Add a few drops of vinegar to eliminate any hidden insects during the final rinse. Drain the greens in a colander.

- **Boiling:** Use a large pot for cooking. For 1 to 1.5 kg of wild greens, you'll need about 3 liters of water. Bring the water to a rolling boil, then add salt and submerge the greens with a fork, ensuring they are well-covered. Stir occasionally. Wild greens need more boiling time than cultivated ones, *approximately 10 minutes*, depending on your preference for tenderness.

- **Serving:** If you enjoy them hot, traditionally served with their broth, place them directly in a bowl with some broth, olive oil, and lemon. This method yields greens with a deep, dark color. For a different serving style, place bread slices on a deep plate, pour over the broth, add some greens on top, drizzle with olive oil and lemon juice, and, finally, add a pinch of salt.

- **Preservation:** To keep boiled horta green, transfer them immediately from the boiling saltwater to a basin filled with ice water. This sudden cooling helps keep their vibrant green color. Always cook with an open pot, as covering makes them darken. Pour lemon juice at the last moment to avoid oxidation. Leftover boiled greens *can be stored in the fridge, covered, for up to three days*. Fresh greens can be stored *on the countertop, covered, for a day.*

- **Freezing raw horta:** Clean raw greens of dirt, roots, and dry leaves for later use, then divide them into bags. They should be *moisture-free before freezing* unless cooked to be used for pies or pasties. In such cases, cut into large pieces, squeeze out moisture, and then freeze in flat shapes for quick defrosting. Properly stored, horta will maintain best quality for about 12 months in the freezer.

56 Types of Horta You'll Find in Crete

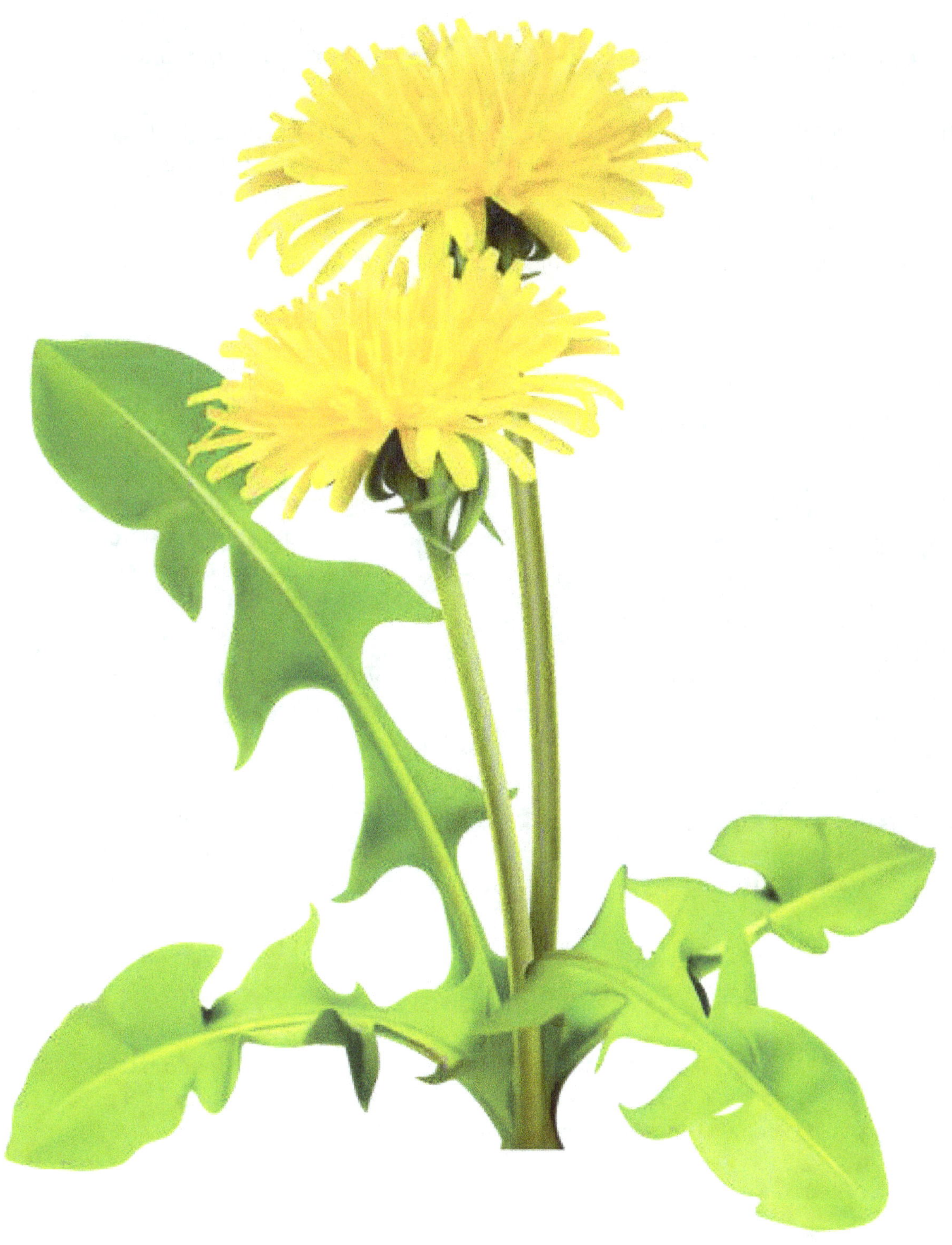

15 - 94

Agoglossos (Anchusa azurea)

Anchusa azurea, a flowering species within the Boraginaceae family, is known by various names, including garden anchusa and Italian bugloss. In Crete, it is referred to as **Agoglossos**.

This herbaceous perennial typically grows to a height of 30-100 cm. The plant features an upright, highly branched stem with long, slender subdivisions. Its lance-shaped leaves extend outward with small toothed edges and are covered with coarse hairs, similar to the stems. The flowers present in shades of blue or pink, measuring 10-12 mm in diameter, and group together in clusters of 3-5 forming a crown-like pattern with five petals, blooming from March to May. Its fruit is small, oval, and slightly tilted.

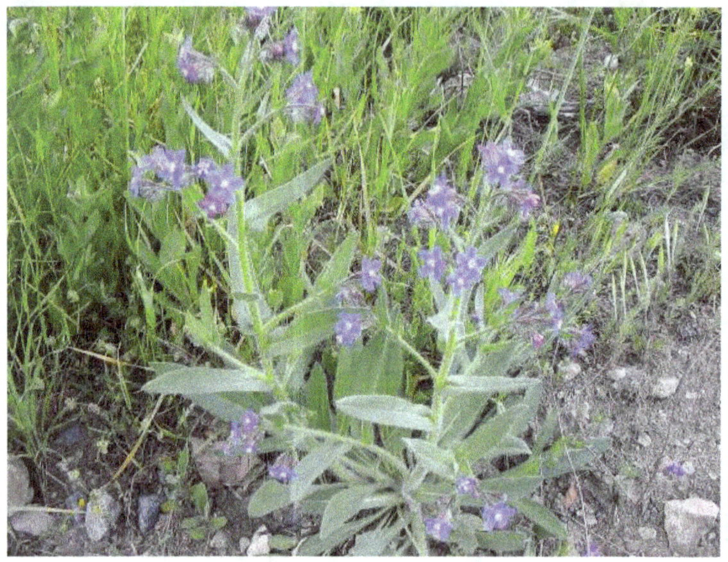

Agoglossos thrives near roadsides in well-drained, nutrient-rich soils, found mainly in lowland and hilly areas. It is rich in vitamin E and contains terpenes and flavonoids. The young, tender leaves are edible and enjoyed for their taste **from March to April (before the first blossoms).**

These leaves are often boiled and served with olive oil and lemon alongside other greens, making a delightful salad.

They can also be cooked and fashioned into meatballs known as **Agoglossokeftedes**. The upper portions of the plant are consumed just after harvesting, preceding flowering, and prepared by boiling and frying in batter.

The plant boasts antibacterial, antioxidant, antitussive, laxative, diaphoretic, and diuretic effects. Dried and ground, it is used as a poultice to reduce inflammation. Studies suggest it has a significant anticancer impact on certain types of cancer cells.

Agriagginara (Cynara cornigera)

Agriagginara, also known as wild artichoke, is a hardy perennial plant notable for its robust and elevated root system and upright stem, which features deep grooves and can grow up to two meters tall. The basal leaves are large, deeply lobed, and vary from light green to yellow-green. Positioned in a scattered pattern, these lance-shaped leaves grow opposite each other. Each leaf is compound, with a clear central vein and distinct spiny sections. The plant's flowers develop from the points where leaves attach to the stem and end in ovoid clusters. These tubular, hermaphroditic flowers bloom profusely from May onwards. The plant produces fruits with numerous seeds, each adorned with several fine hairs.

This species flourishes in low-altitude regions with shrubs and rocky surfaces, managing well in nutrient-poor soils, whether acidic or alkaline. It needs at least 350-400 mm of annual rainfall. While its foliage emerges in early spring, the plant blooms later.

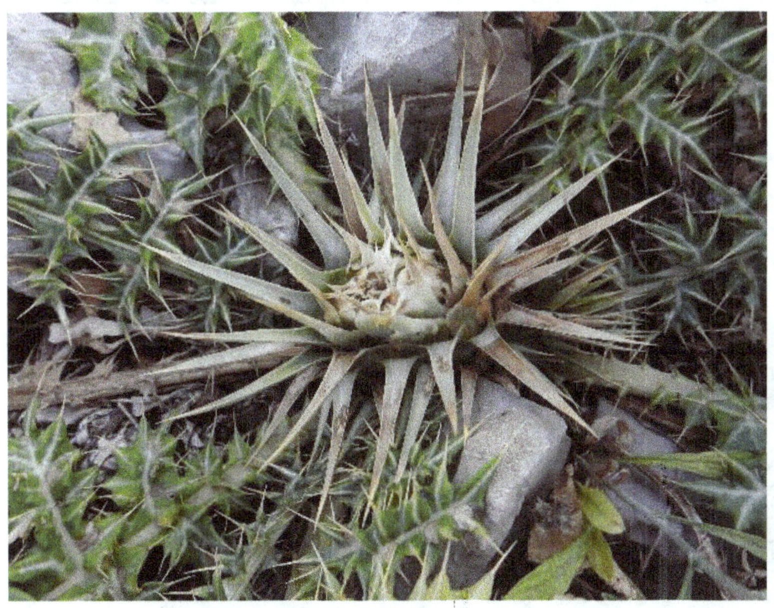

The wild artichoke is rich in calcium, phosphate, vitamins, organic acids, and compounds like quinarin and inulin.

Young shoots, as well as stalks and leaves, are edible after being trimmed and cooked. A popular dish includes egg-lemon fricassee with meat, such as lamb, goat, or fish. The floral buds are also prepared with scrambled eggs or preserved through pickling.

Wild artichoke benefits health by stimulating bile production, reducing urea levels, decreasing blood cholesterol, lowering blood pressure, and alleviating prostate enlargement. A decoction made from leaves and petals helps treat fever; one or two cups are suggested daily. Fresh leaves, when crushed, serve as an effective poultice for hemorrhoids. Poultices of boiled leaves left overnight can treat tonsillitis and sore throats.

Ágrio spanáki (Rhagadiolus edulis)

Ágrio spanáki, also known as wild spinach or edible star-hawkbit, is an annual plant with slender stems that spread out along the ground or grow partly upright, reaching up to 50 centimeters. Its leaves are attached directly to the stem, with jagged margins that are larger at the base and become smaller and more narrow toward the tip.

The plant features small yellow flowers surrounded by eight bracts, each with a fine layer of tiny hairs. Its fruit is an achene, slightly curved inward. This plant thrives in shaded areas, often found beneath shrubs, within olive groves, and in well-moisturized soil with high clay content, especially **during spring.**

The plant's tissues contain flavonoids like quercetin, luteolin, and nicotiflorin, along with phenolic acids such as 3,5-dicaffeoylquinic acid and chlorogenic acid, and other active compounds. **Before flowering**, the young leaves and shoots are edible and typically incorporated into dishes like tsigariastá (sauteed horta) or kalitsoúnia (pies), mixed with various other greens.

Ágrio spanáki is known for its antioxidant and antibacterial qualities.

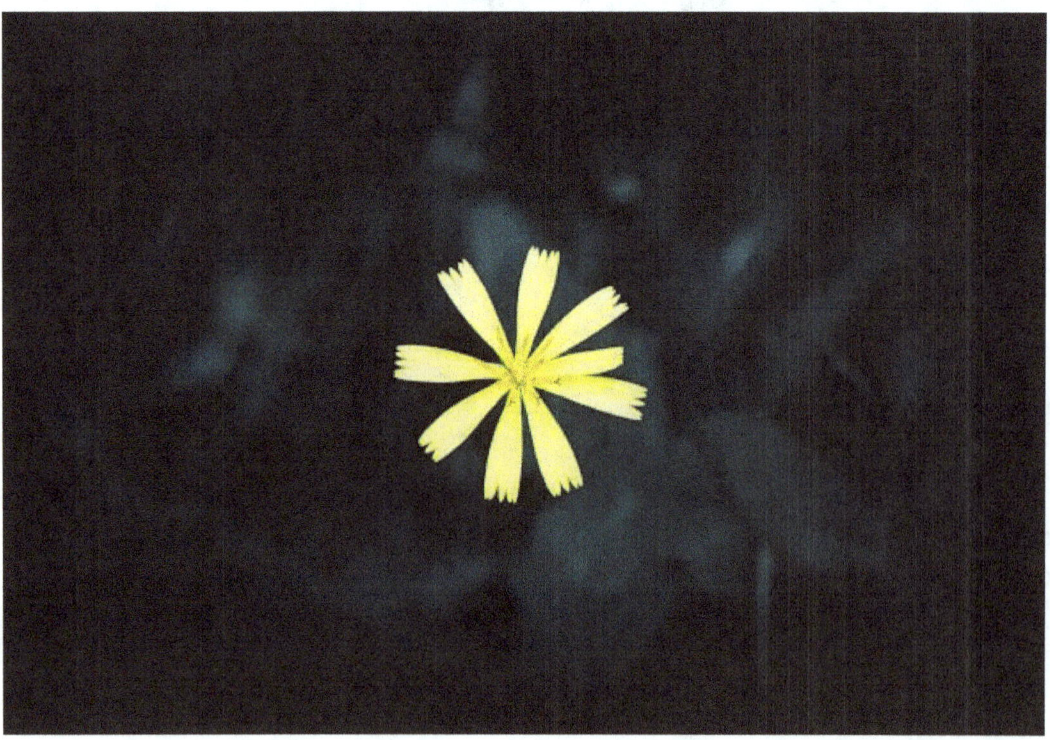

Photo by Wyxina Tresse

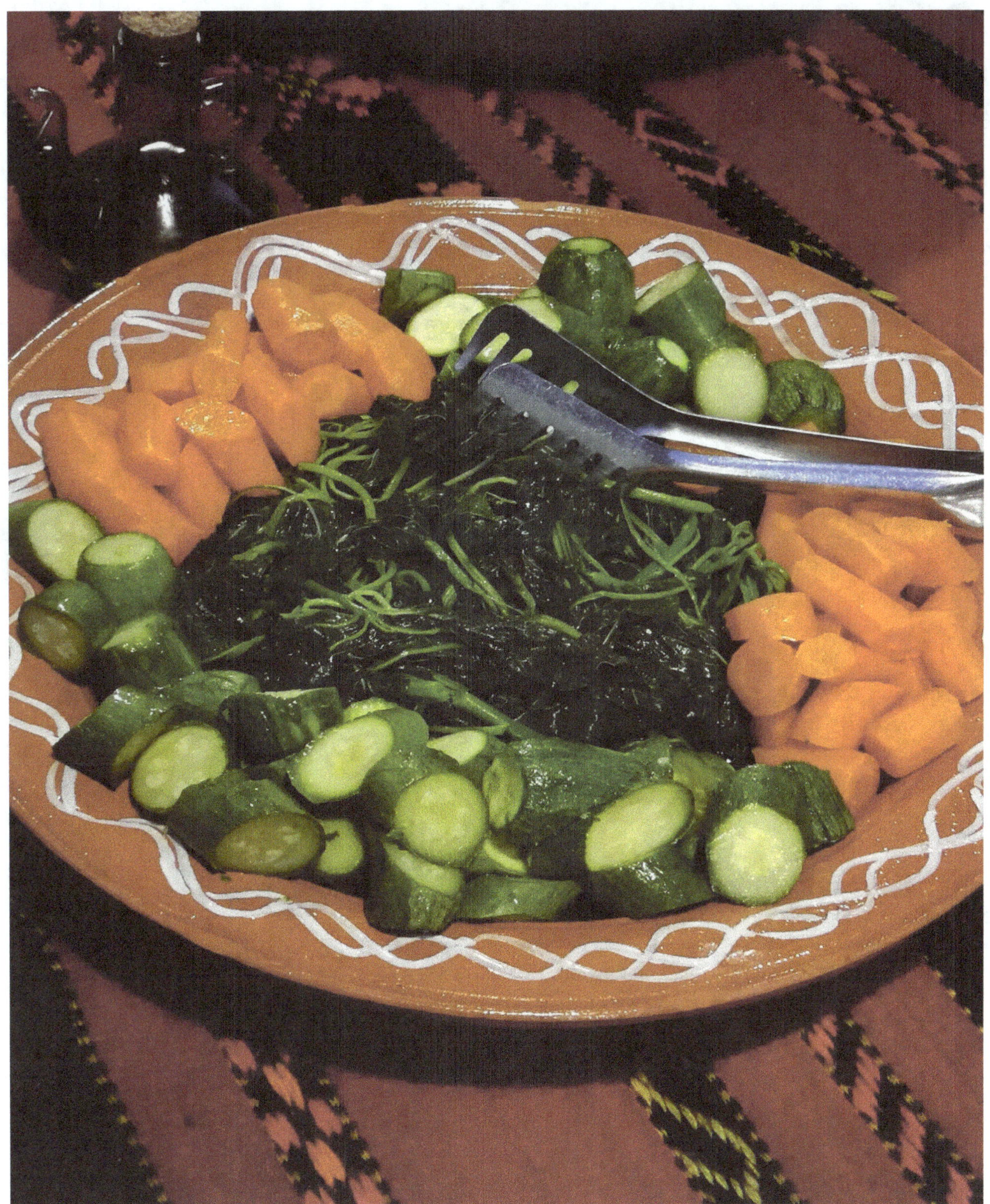

Boiled horta vlita with boiled carrots and zucchini.

Agriovrouva (Sisymbrium officinale)

Sisymbrium officinale, commonly called hedge mustard or agriovrouva in Greek, is an annual plant with a hairy texture. It features a strong, upright stem, reaching heights between 25 and 60 centimeters, with lateral branches. Its leaves alternate along the stem; the lower ones possess a serrated, feather-like appearance, while the upper ones are lance-shaped.

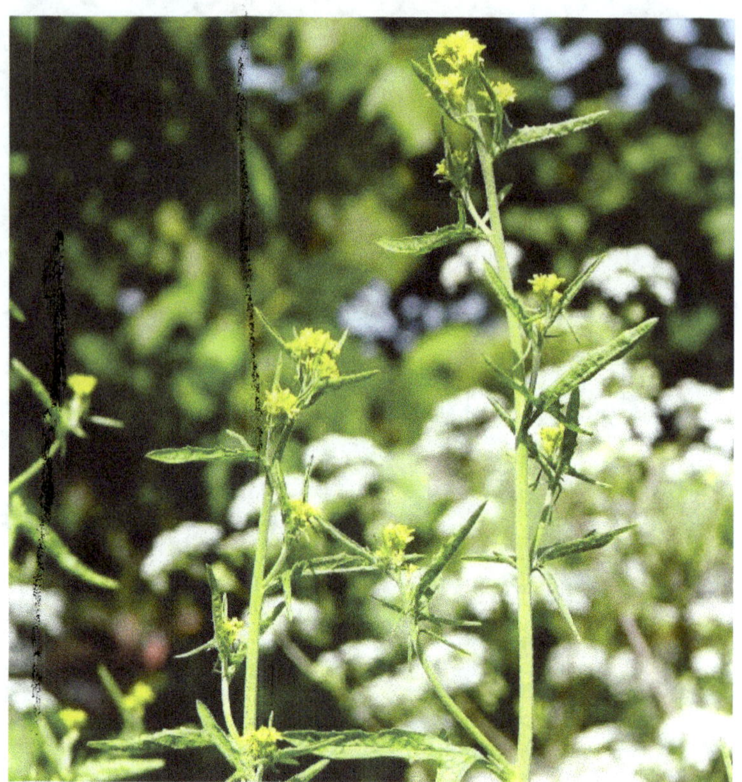

The small, pale yellow flowers are hermaphroditic and form clusters, blossoming from February to September. The pubescent fruit tapers to a narrow tip. This plant flourishes in sunlit, chalky soils. It is often found in both farmed and wild fields, along roadsides, on poor or silty ground, and even among waste. It contains sulfur compounds and cardenolides.

The piquant leaves and tender stems, **harvested in winter and spring**, are enjoyed raw or cooked. They add flavor to salads, vegetable pies, and rich dishes.

Hedge mustard has several beneficial properties, including laxative, detoxifying, antibacterial, expectorant, astringent, diuretic, and tonic qualities. Its fruit extract, containing a high level of cardenolides, benefits the cardiovascular system.

Photo by Evelyn Simak

Agriolláchano (Brassica cretica subsp. aegaea)

Agriolláchano—the **wild cabbage**—scientifically referred to as Brassica cretica (subsp. aegaea), is a perennial herb distinguished by its branching stems that emerge from the base, reaching up to 1.2 meters in height.

The plant features large, elongated, succulent leaves with minimal hairs along the edges, displaying a bright green color. Its flowers, grouped in dense vertical clusters, bloom in a striking yellow from March through early June. It flourishes in calcareous rocky soils that drain well and receive ample sunlight, particularly those facing north and thrives at elevations between sea level and 1,000 meters.

Often, agriolláchano inhabits canyons and undisturbed limestone slopes within ravines. Agriolláchano is a rich source of vitamin K, vitamin O, and calcium, all essential for maintaining healthy bones. It also contains vitamins A and B. **The tender shoots and leaves** are typically harvested in spring and consumed after boiling, often served in salads seasoned with olive oil. Known for its health benefits,

Agriolláchano possesses laxative, antiseptic, anti-inflammatory, anti-hemorrhagic, and potential anti-cancer properties.

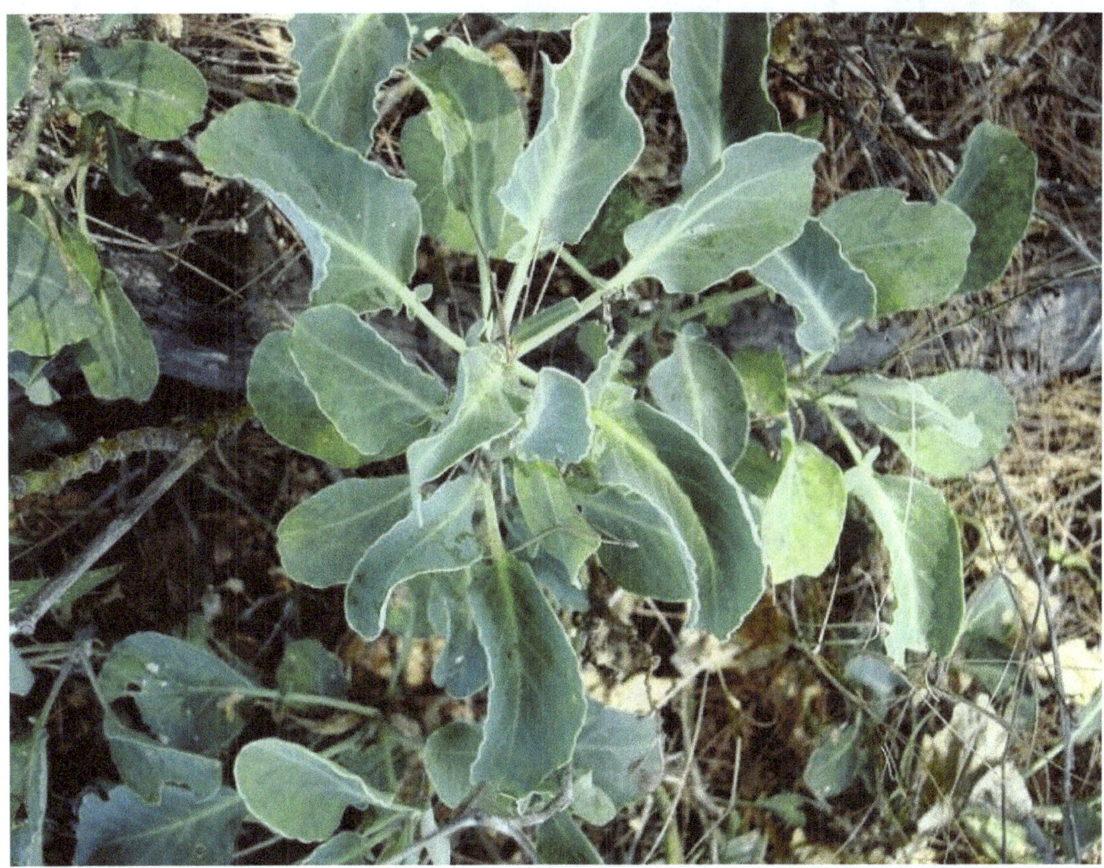

Photo by
Stavros Apostolou

Agrios Maïntanós (Scaligeria napiformis—syn. Scaligeria cretica)

Agrios maïntanós, the wild parsley, is a biennial plant notable for its spindle-shaped tuberous root. Its stem stands upright, smooth, and cylindrical, branching out with a greenish-red hue, reaching heights of 15 to 50 cm.

The plant's leaves are intricately shaped, featuring multiple leaflets that form a feather-like pattern with diamond or egg-shaped segments and tooth-like edges. The upper leaves are narrower and lance-shaped. Its white flowers form in umbrella-like clusters of 5 to 25 rays of different lengths, typically blooming from April to May. The fruit is characterized by its dichotomous nature.

Wild parsley flourishes on terraced, rocky, less fertile lands, shaded regions with adequate rainfall, and clay-rich areas in semi-mountainous zones. It becomes available for consumption from February to April.

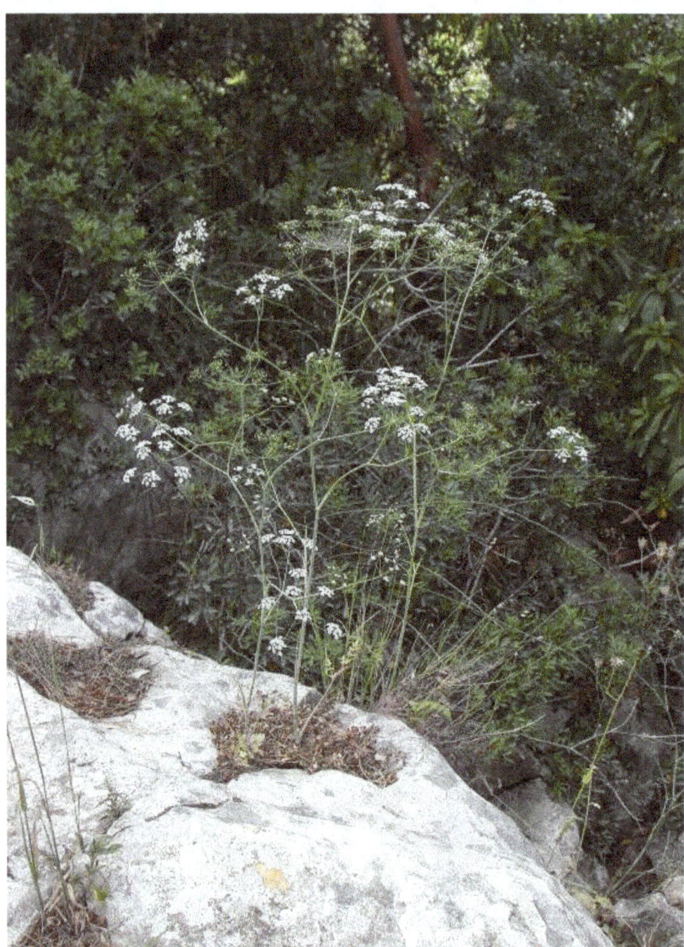

Scaligeria cretica is rich in vitamins A, C, E, B12, and K, along with β-carotene, folic acid, and minerals like calcium, magnesium, iron, phosphorus, potassium, and manganese.

Young branches and leaves are **harvested before flowering**. Known for its strong aroma and sweet and flavorful taste, agrios maïntanós is often paired with other seasonal herbs in dishes like sizzling greens, herb pies, and kalitsounia.Agrios maïntanós offers anti-inflammatory properties, acts as a diuretic, and boosts the immune system.

Its richvitamin C and iron composition also helps fight anemia and fatigue.

Photo by Gideon Pisanty

Agriópraso (Allium ampeloprasum)

Agriópraso, the wild leek, is a perennial plant featuring a bulbous T-root and a smooth, sturdy stem that usually reaches 50 to 100 centimeters in height. Its leaves are long, grooved, and slender, with jagged edges near the base. Atop a sleek, hollow stem that can stretch up to one meter, the flower emerges through a thin sheath. The floral arrangement is umbellate, showcasing numerous small purple blooms between May and June.

This plant flourishes best in sunny, moist locations, such as meadows and cultivated or abandoned fields in lowland and semi-mountainous regions. It prefers well-drained soils with a medium texture, rich in organic matter, and a pH between 6 and 7. Rich in vitamins A, B, and C and packed with minerals like potassium, magnesium, and zinc, as well as other antioxidant compounds, the plant's delicate stem and bulb are **harvested from February to May**.

It is frequently combined with other foraged greens and used in dishes like stews, pies, and kalitsounia. It is often cooked with rice or added to meat pies to enhance flavor. It pairs well with celery or tomato due to its garlicky aroma and appealing taste.

Agriópraso possesses diuretic properties and can help treat skin conditions such as burns and respiratory issues like coughs and arthritis.

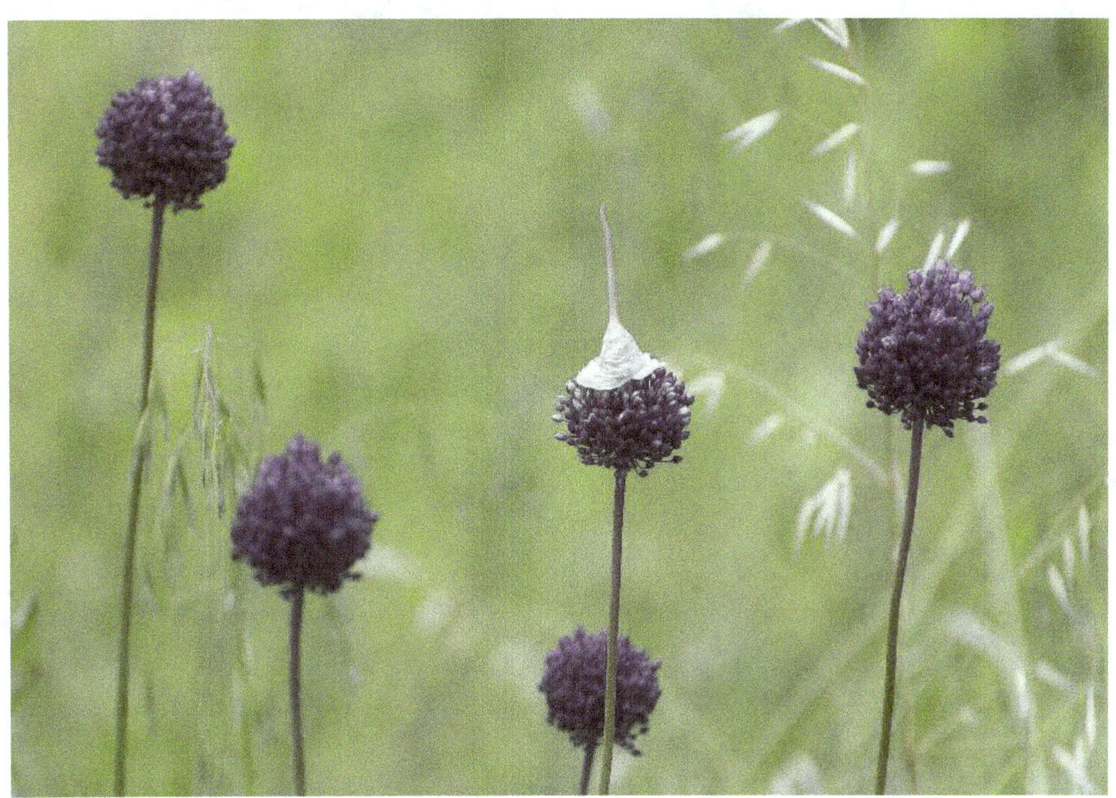

Photo by Pit56

Agriosélino (Apium nodiflorum)

Agriosélino—wild celery—scientifically known as Apium nodiflorum, is a perennial plant notable for its smooth, hollow, and often angular stems. It typically reaches heights between 30 and 80 cm. The plant's leaves are sleek, featuring 2 to 8 pairs of serrated leaflets. Its small, white flowers form in terminal clusters and bloom from July to August. The fruit of wild celery is small, about 2 millimeters long, and dark brown with an oblong shape.

This plant thrives in wetland environments, including marshes, streams, rivers, and other moist areas. Wild celery is abundant in calcium, salt, and oxalic acid. It also provides substantial amounts of vitamins C, E, and B9, along with phenolic compounds and flavonoids, primarily quercetin.

Young shoots and leaves harvested in the months before the plant blooms are valued for their fragrance in culinary uses. They are often used in fried dishes or as an ingredient in pies, sometimes mixed with other greens. This plant is known to stimulate appetite and reduce inflammation in the digestive system. It also displays diuretic, antibacterial, and antifungal properties.

Due to its high oxalic acid content, those with liver issues should **consume it in moderation.**

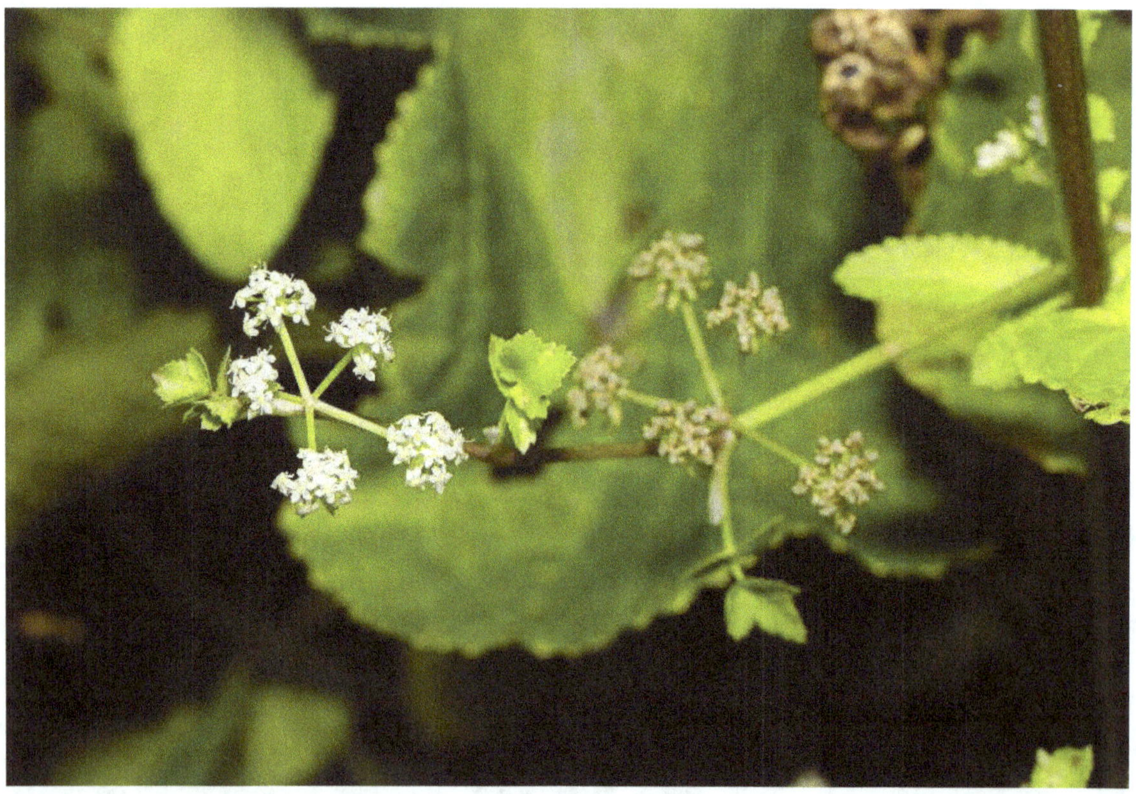

Photo by Stephen James

McWilliam

Akournópodas (Oenanthe pimpinelloides)

Akournópoda—in English, corky-fruited water-dropwort and known scientifically as *Oenanthe pimpinelloides*—is a perennial plant notable for its bluish-green leaves. The plant's base presents pinnate leaves with wide ovate or lanceolate shapes and serrated edges.

By late March, a tall, woody stem grows from the center, topped with white flowers resembling small, clear umbrellas. These flowers appear between May and June.

Akournópoda flourishes in uncultivated fields and marshy areas with moderate rainfall, particularly in lowland, hilly, and semi-valley regions, thriving best in acidic soil under ample rainfall. Its optimal growth period is from early January to late March. **From January to March**, the plant's leaves and stems are harvested for consumption.

They are typically prepared by boiling, frying, or fricasseeing, often combined with other leafy greens. These parts are also useful in dishes like pies and kalitsounia. When paired with salted cod, they create a delightful stew. Other corky-fruited water-dropwort stew options include pork or goat, yet they remain just as tasty when cooked with chicken or cuttlefish.

Rich in minerals like calcium, potassium, sodium, iron, magnesium, phosphorus, and zinc, Akournópoda offers nutritional benefits. It also contains vitamin C, beta-carotene, and vitamin A.

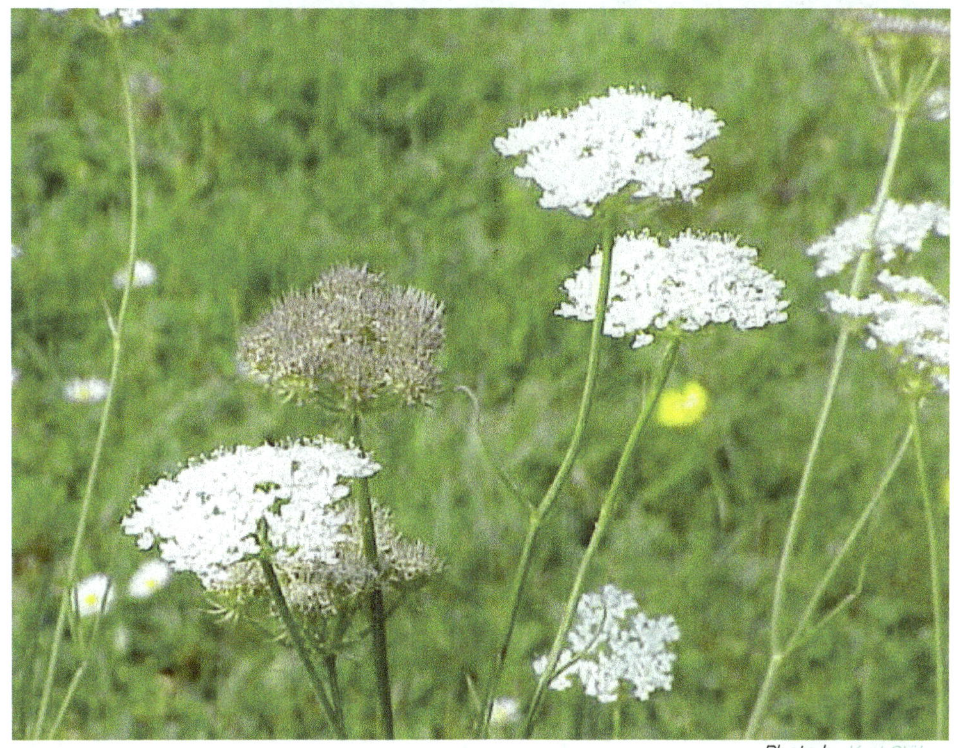

Photo by Kurt Stüber.

Amáranto (Limonium sinuatum)

Amáranto, in English, wavyleaf sea lavender, is a perennial herbaceous plant notable for its slender, leafless stem, which reaches heights between 40 and 60 cm. The stem is sturdy, roughly square, and features distinct linear wings covered in tough hairs. The leaves originate from the plant's base, forming circular rosettes. These leaves range from 5 to 20 cm long and have serrated edges.

The plant produces flower clusters from March to June at the top of its stems. These clusters, or corymbs, contain flowers with both male and female parts, showcasing white petals with purple-violet calyxes. Amáranto adapts well to poor, sandy, and rocky coastal soils, enduring arid climates and growing at altitudes up to 450 meters.

The **tender leaves, young stems, and rosettes harvested in spring** are edible after boiling and are often added to salads, either alone or with other greens. They also make an excellent addition to fish dishes, couscous, and even rich vegetable soups and risottos.

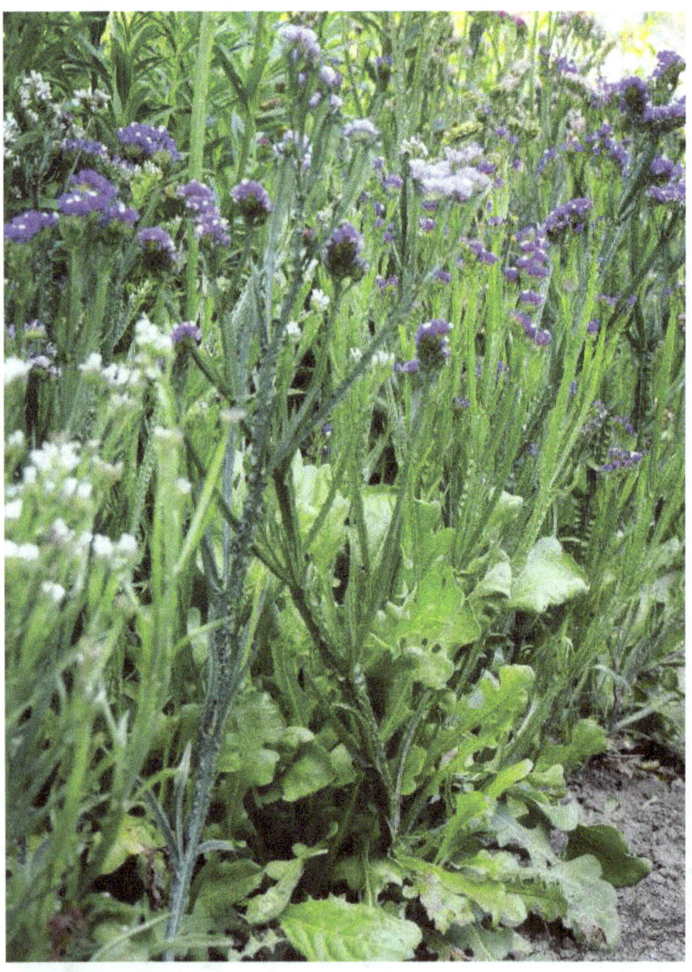

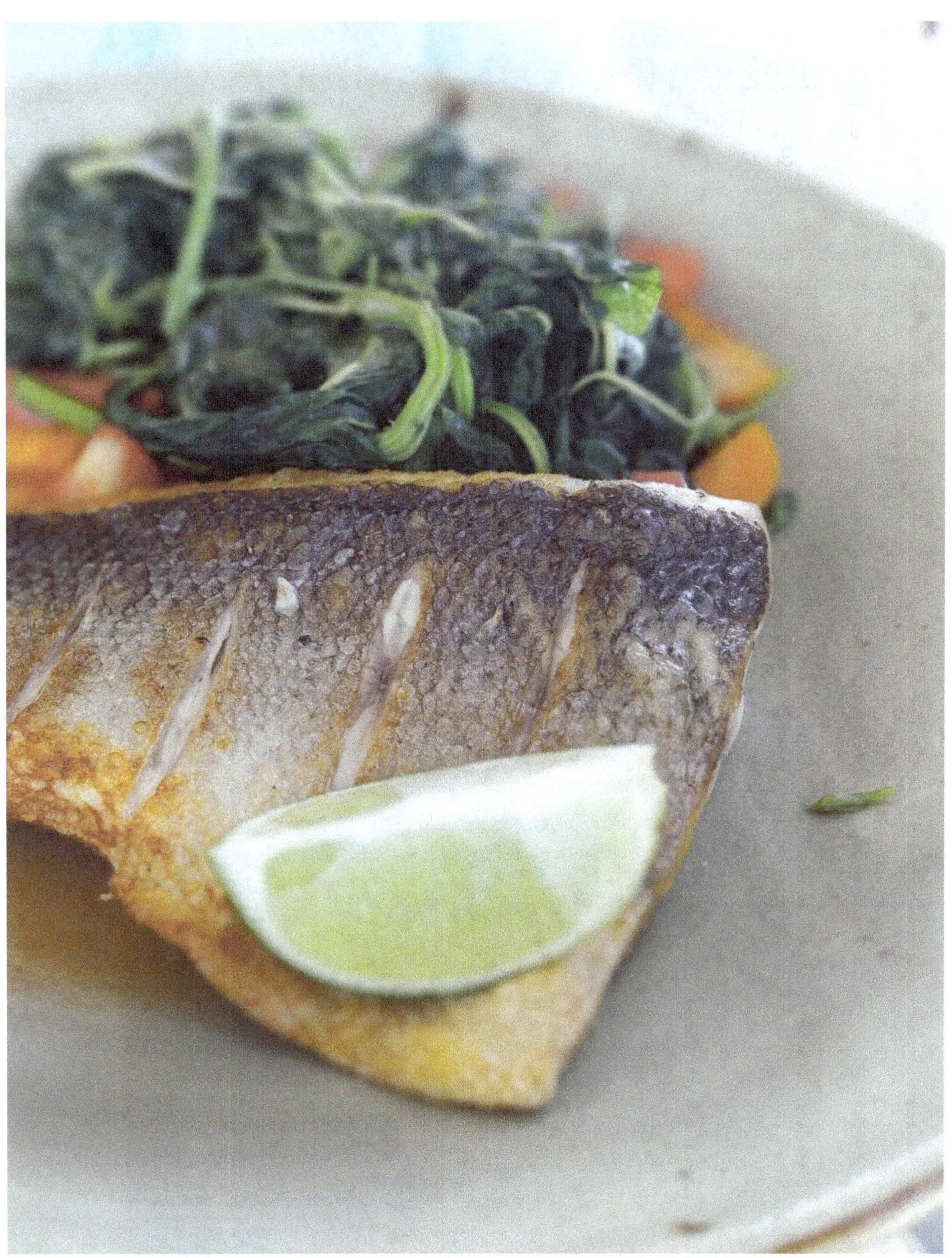

Many horta varieties, especially the leafy ones, pair well with fish.

Ascordulakas (Muscari comosum)

Ascordulakas—in English, wild tassel hyacinth (Muscari comosum)—is a perennial plant with a firm stem reaching about 15 to 50 centimeters. This plant does not have leaves along its stem. Three to seven folded leaves appear near the base, arranged along their central vein.

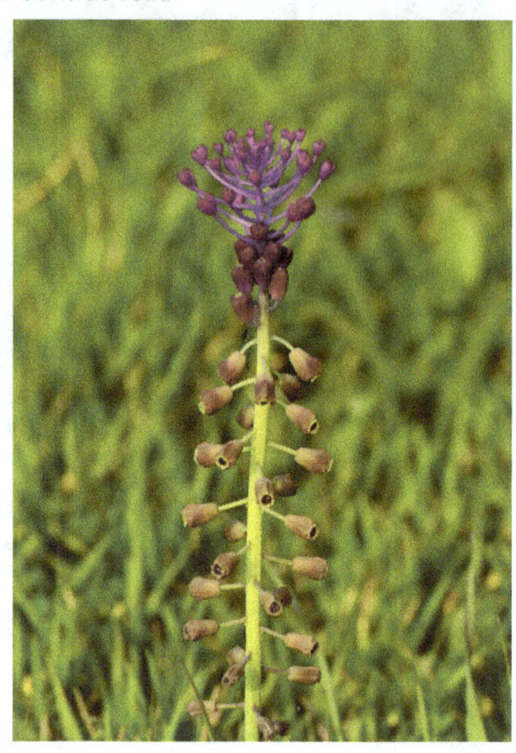

At the stem's tip, it forms a cluster of flowers. The lower blooms are fertile with a bell shape and pale lobes, while the infertile blossoms at the top are blue-violet and plume-like. It blooms in late spring or summer, depending on location. The fruit develops as pyramid-like capsules filled with numerous small seeds.

Ascordulakas prospers in low-altitude areas with rocky, well-drained soils. It's found in hills and cultivated or abandoned fields. The bulbs lie underground and are **collected from April to May**, easily identified by their distinct flower cluster.

These bulbs contain starch, glysmatic elements, fatty acids (notably with a strong ω6/ω3 ratio), pentosans, vitamins A and C, cellulose, phosphate, and calcium. They are prepared by boiling and pickling with vinegar, dill, and onion, serving as appetizers—a Cretan specialty known as Pickled Volvoi / Βολβοί Τουρσί. Sprouts and flowers can be smoked or added to omelets.

The pink Volvoi taste bitter but are considered higher quality, so they will be more expensive in supermarkets, whereas the white bulbs are sweeter but less desirable and are cheaper.

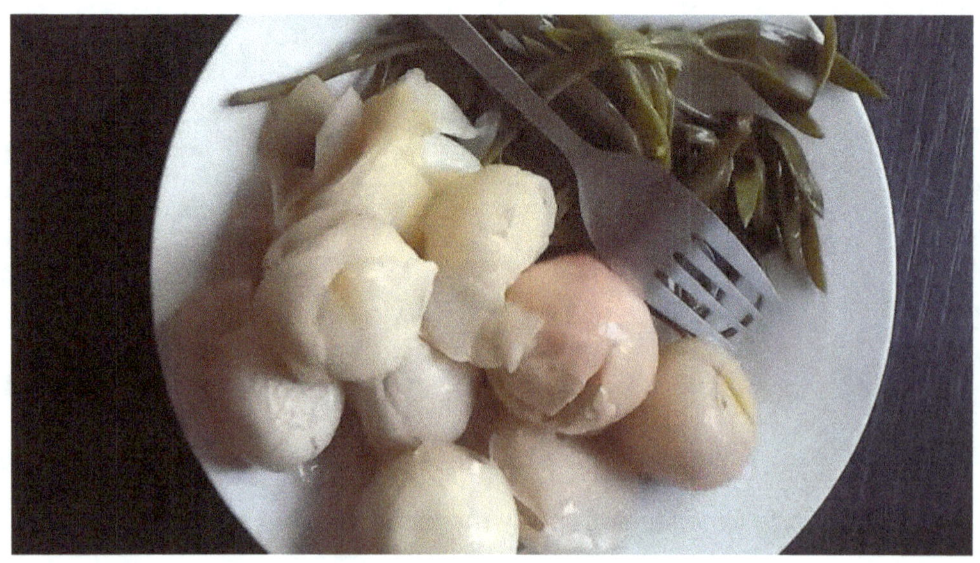

Askordoúlakas áspros (Ornithogalum narbonense)

Ornithogalum narbonense, commonly referred to as Narbonne star-of-Bethlehem and askordoúlakas áspros in Greek, is a hardy perennial plant known for its large oval-shaped bulb and straight stem reaching 40 to 80 centimeters.

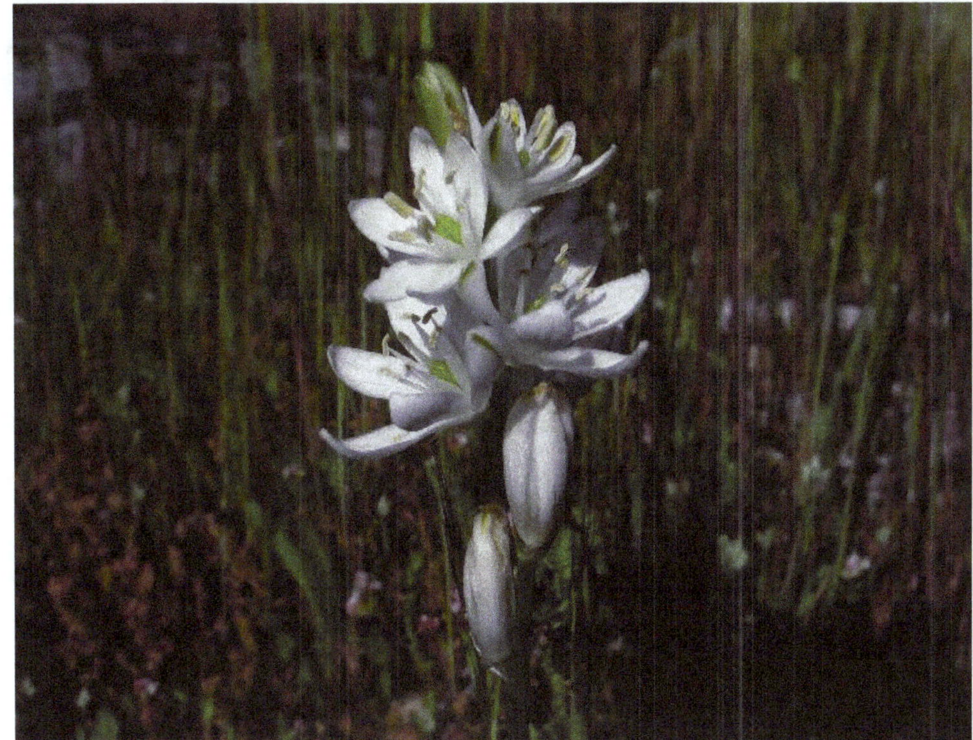

Typically, this plant forms a rosette of 4-6 leaves, which are simple, narrow, and have parallel edges without any hair. The flowers display a milky-white color with a green line beneath. They form a loose cluster, holding between 20 to 50 individual blooms.

Askordoúlakas áspros blooms from late March through early June. The fruit appears as a capsule divided into sections. It thrives on rocky slopes and field edges, including uncultivated areas and wheat fields, up to elevations of 1200 meters.

The identifiable bulbs hide underground and are **collectible from April to May**, distinguished by their singular floral arrangement.

The bulbs boast starchy and glycemic substances, healthy fatty acids with an excellent ω6/ω3 ratio, pentosans, vitamins A and C, cellulose, phosphate, and calcium.

Locals boil the bulbs and then pickle them with vinegar, dill, and onion, creating a flavorful appetizer. Sprouts with their flowers can be smoked or added to omelettes. Although white bovids have a more pleasant taste, they are considered of lower quality. Bulb extracts exhibit strong antioxidant and blood sugar-lowering properties.

Ascolympros (Scolymus hispanicus)

Ascolympros (Scolymus hispanicus)—the common golden thistle or Spanish oyster thistle—offers edible parts ideal for culinary use. After removing the thorns, both the foliage and the inner root bark can be used.

They are often boiled and served solo as a salad or mixed with other greens. Another option is to cook them with rice. They pair deliciously in fricassee dishes with egg-lemon sauce and either pork or fish. The roots are also boiled before consumption.

This hardy perennial plant is notable for its strong taproot and central stem that branches with thorny edges. When cut, the root and stem release a milky sap.

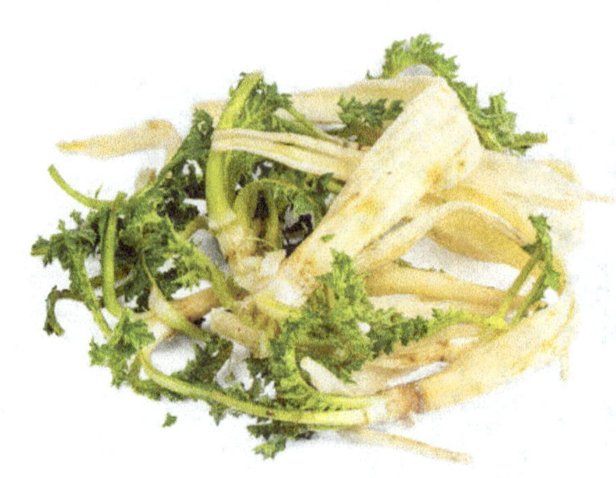

The leaves, growing from the base, are tender, shaped like a lance, with occasional spines and long stems. Its flowers emerge from leaf junctions, forming clusters of numerous yellow blossoms.

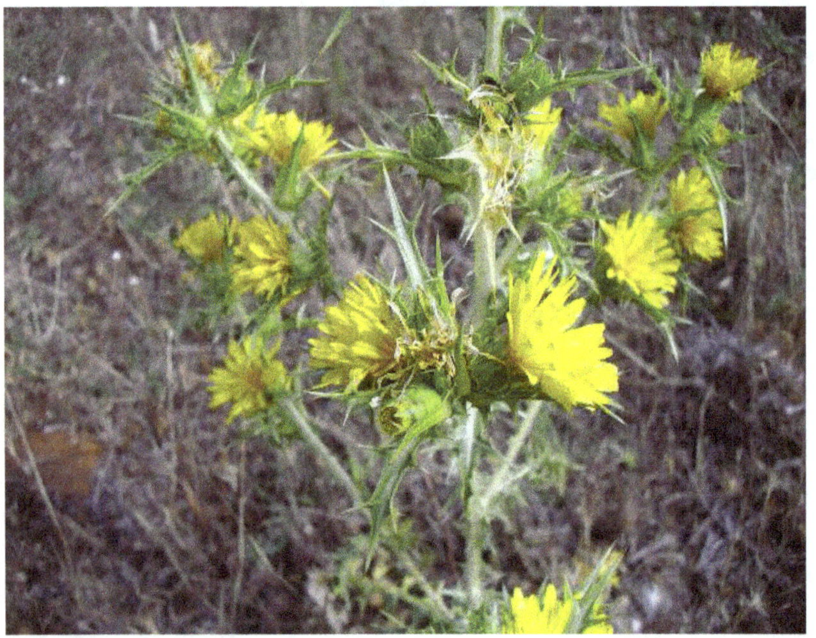

Ascolympros thrives well in cultivated and wild fields during winter and spring across various environments, from hillsides to coastal areas. The plant is rich in vitamins K, O, and β-carotene, alongside proteins, chlorophyll, and flavonoids.

People enjoy it as spungato (omelet) or after marinating it in vinegar and preserving it in olive oil, making it an excellent appetizer or complement to ouzo or Cretan raki (tsikoudia, a type of grape pomace brandy).

The plant is known to benefit gastrointestinal issues, skin conditions, kidney stones, and arthritis. The remaining water from the boiled root is consumed as a herbal tea for its medicinal benefits.

Chátzikas (Scandix pecten veneris L.)

Chátzikas, also known as shepherd's-needle or Venus' comb, is a perennial herb noted for its soft texture and marked stem, reaching 10 to 30 centimeters. Its root resembles a stilt and is not deeply embedded. The plant features small, serrated leaves that grow in pairs and consist of 3 to 9 finely divided leaflets, each separated into distinct lobes.

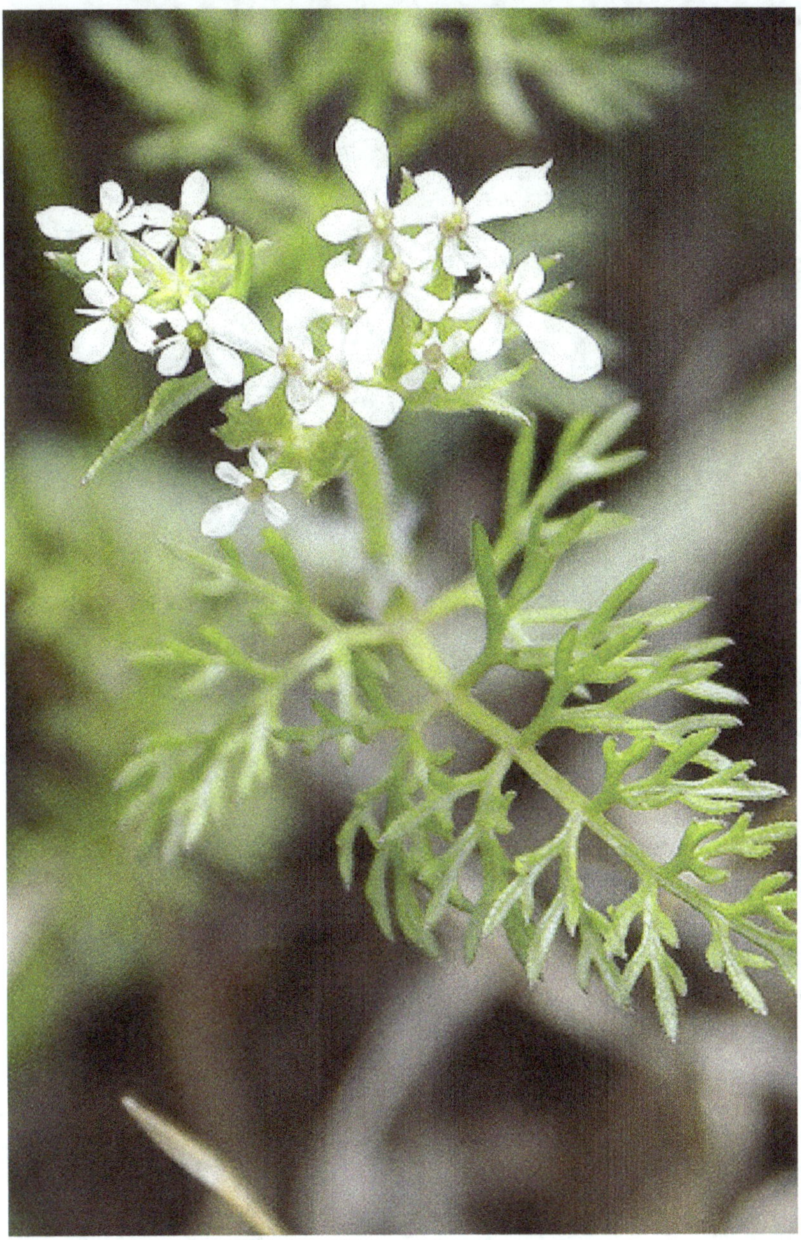

This edible green produces white flowers, grouped into clusters of 2 to 3 rays, appearing in spring near the top of the stems. The plant's fruit is elongated, spanning 1 to 4 centimeters, with a beak matching the seed section in length. It adapts well to wild and farmed soils and grows in meadows. It often lines roadsides in lowland and foothill regions.

Chátzikas is rich in nutrients such as α-tocopherol, β-carotene, potassium, sodium, phosphorus, iron, magnesium, manganese, and zinc. Due to its fragrance and unique taste, chátzikas is an ingredient in dishes like vegetable pies, kalitsounias, omelets, and fried greens. It also complements meat, fish, and legumes while being a flavorful addition to soups or steamed, served as a warm salad.

Known for its medicinal properties, chátzikas offers anti-inflammatory, expectorant, diuretic, tonic, and laxative benefits. Traditionally, its decoction has been used to treat dyspepsia, cystitis, gastroenteritis, nephritis, and pyelitis. Moreover, it is highly appreciated for its stimulating and aphrodisiac effects.

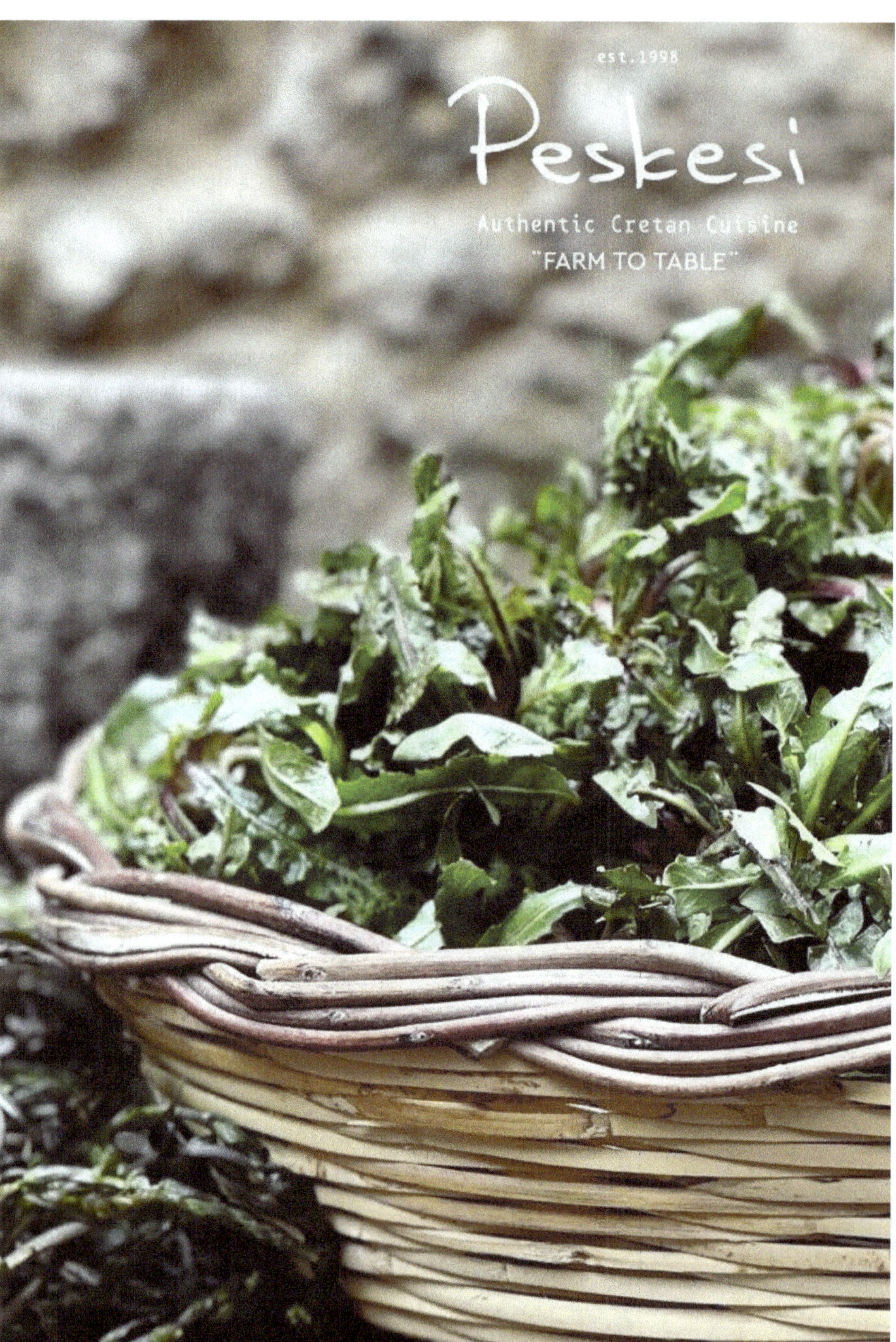

Peskesi is one of the best destinations in Heraklion for seasonal horta.

Chinopódio (Chenopodiastrum murale)

Chenopodiastrum murale—nettle-leaved goosefoot, Australian-spinach, salt-green, and sowbane—in Greek as Chinopódio, is an annual plant usually growing to a height of 1 to 70 cm, often displaying either red or green streaks on its stem.

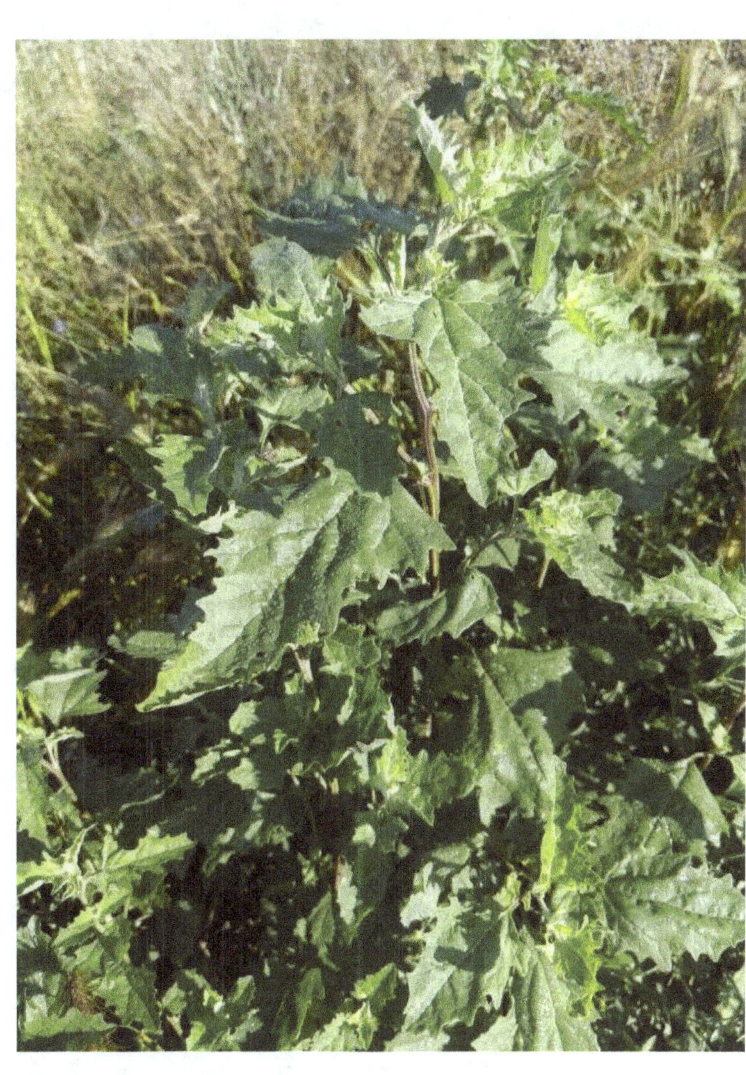

The leaves are shaped oval to triangular with jagged edges, wide in size. On the upper side, the leaves feel smooth, while the underside appears with a yellowish hue.

The plant's flowers cluster in dense groups of tiny spherical buds. This hermaphroditic species blooms from July to October, with seeds ripening from August to October.

This plant can adapt to various soil types, ranging from light to heavy clay, acidic or alkaline, regardless of nutrient content. While it flourishes in moist soil, it can also endure dry conditions.

Chinopódio contains oxalic acid and saponins, toxic substances that are generally minimal and removed through cooking.

The leaves and young shoots can be consumed raw or cooked, much like spinach, but only in limited quantities due to their toxic nature.

Choiromourída (Helminthotheca echioides)

Choiromourída—bristly (or prickly) oxtongue—known scientifically as Helminthotheca echioides, is a prickly perennial weed. It grows with an upright stem that can reach up to 1 meter in height and features numerous branches covered in stiff hairs.

The plant's leaves are long, tough, serrated, and have tiny pale blisters, with the stem displaying wing-like extensions. Its flowers bloom between **March and May**, exhibiting a pale yellow color in their tongue-shaped heads. The fruit produced is a type of achene with a pointed beak.

This plant usually grows in cultivated fields, particularly in lowland and semi-mountainous areas. It favors environments with higher moisture levels and often flourishes near grassy regions and along stream banks.

Rich in beneficial compounds, Choiromourída contains flavonoids, phenols, α-tocopherol, and minerals such as potassium, sodium, calcium, iron, magnesium, copper, zinc, manganese, and phosphorus.

Culinary preparation typically involves boiling the plant (mainly the leaves), then straining it and serving it with lemon oil, often paired with other greens like artichokes or courgettes. It is appreciated for its antioxidant, anti-inflammatory, and antibacterial properties. Once dehydrated, it is employed as a poultice to alleviate inflammations.

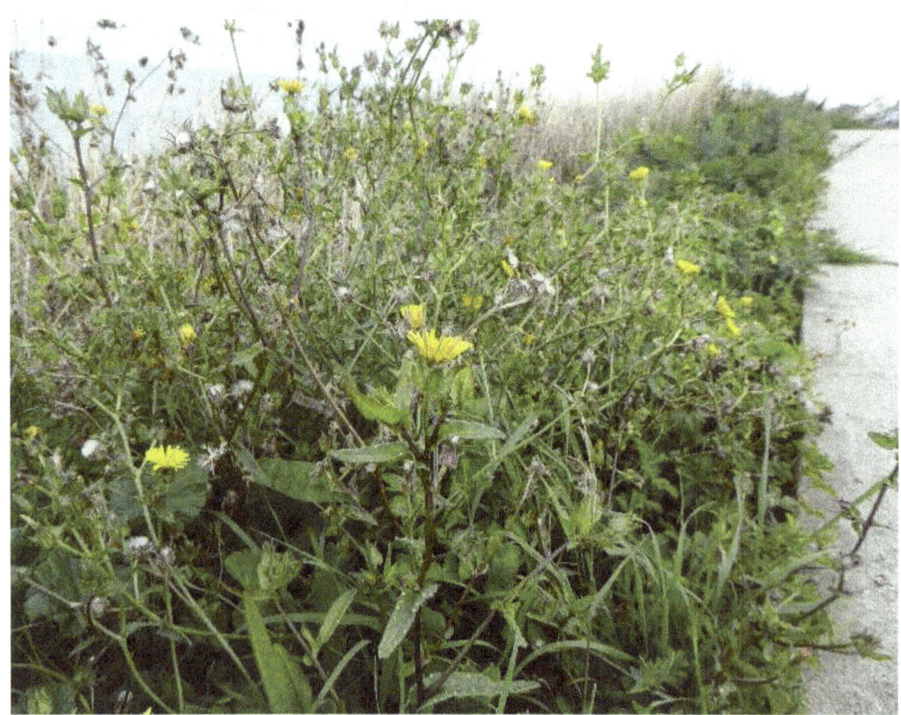

Photo by Alex Lockton

Galatsída (Reichardia picroides)

Galatsída, known scientifically as *Reichardia picroides*, is a perennial herbaceous plant growing between 15 to 40 centimeters tall. It features a supportive stilt base and an upright, branched stem with a subtle blue tone. Its lower leaves exhibit a pinnate design, while the upper leaves have serrated edges and a soft, mushy feel.

The plant's flowers are hermaphroditic, containing both male and female reproductive structures. They form a flower head and display a yellow color, typically blooming from March to May. This plant flourishes in rich soils, both cultivated and wild, and in stony areas.

Harvesting the above-ground parts occurs before the flowering stage, **beginning in October** when it first appears and continuing until just before the blossoms open. The entire plant contains a sticky latex substance. Galatsída is rich in minerals and micronutrients.

A 100-gram portion provides 108 mg of vitamin K, 33 mg of vitamin C, 586 mg of β-carotene, along with various essential minerals such as 3.82 mg of potassium, 448 mg of sodium, 1.55 mg of calcium, 454 mg of magnesium, 41.7 mg of iron, 3.63 mg of copper, 9.98 mg of manganese, 7.01 mg of zinc, and 422 mg of phosphorus.

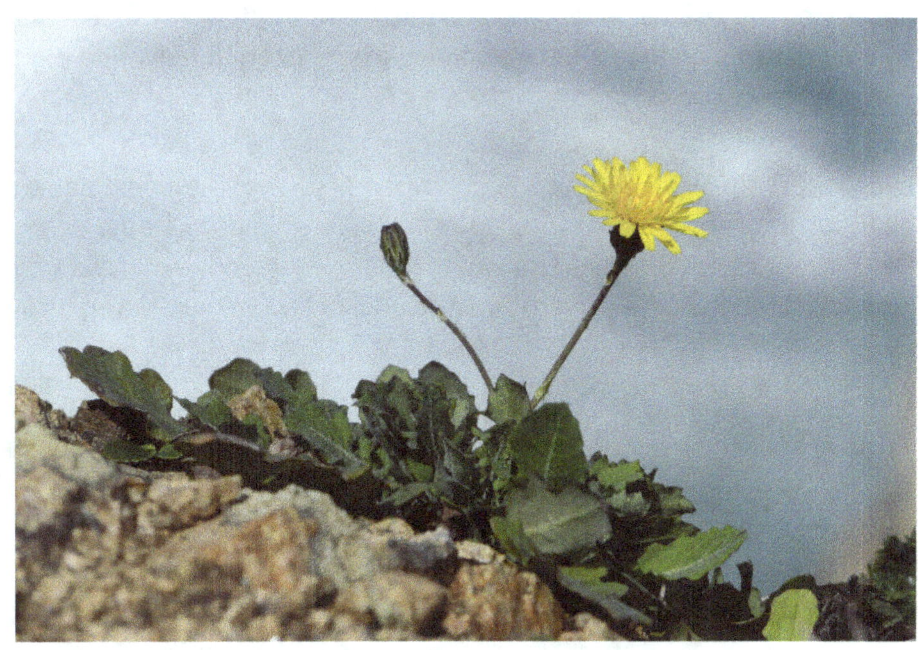

The plant has low nitrite content and contains phenolic compounds like luteolin, apigenin, and chlorogenic acids. Lutein is present, whereas coumarin is absent. It is known for its detoxifying, heart-strengthening, antioxidant, and pain-relieving properties.

Galatsída is edible, both fresh and cooked before it blooms. It has a pleasant aroma and a slightly sweet taste. When raw, it is often used in salads alongside other vegetables. Cooking methods include boiling, stewing, frying, or creating a meat fricassee.

Gérontas (Urospermum picroides)

Urospermum picroides—prickly golden fleece—is packed with nutrients such as vitamin C, polyphenols, flavonoids, omega-3 fatty acids, α-linolenic acid, and essential minerals like phosphorus, magnesium, and iron. The young rosehip leaves are primarily prepared with other vegetables and offer a pleasant, sweet flavor from February to May.

This plant features antioxidant, antibacterial, and anti-inflammatory properties. Its tender shoots are typically consumed to enjoy these benefits. Gérontas is a perennial grass with a deep, simple or branching root system. It has an upright stem that branches out and grows to a height of 30 to 50 cm, covered with fine hairs.

The basal leaves are arranged alternately, simple in structure with a lyre-shaped pinnate form and serrated edges, with sparse hairs along the main veins. They have flat petioles, often purple at the base. The stem leaves are oblong-ovate, without stalks, edged with uneven teeth, having pointed tips, and lobed bases that wrap around the stem. Its flowers appear as yellow florets in terminal and solitary clusters on long stalks, blooming from **March to May**. The plant produces a cylindrical achene fruit with white contents.

Urospermum picroides thrives in cultivated fields, olive groves, barren plains, and along roadsides at altitudes ranging from sea level to 1,200 meters. Once a staple among various wild species used for food, it now remains familiar mainly to older generations and rural communities. In traditional cooking, prickly golden fleece is served raw in salads, boiled with extra virgin olive oil, or cooked in soups.

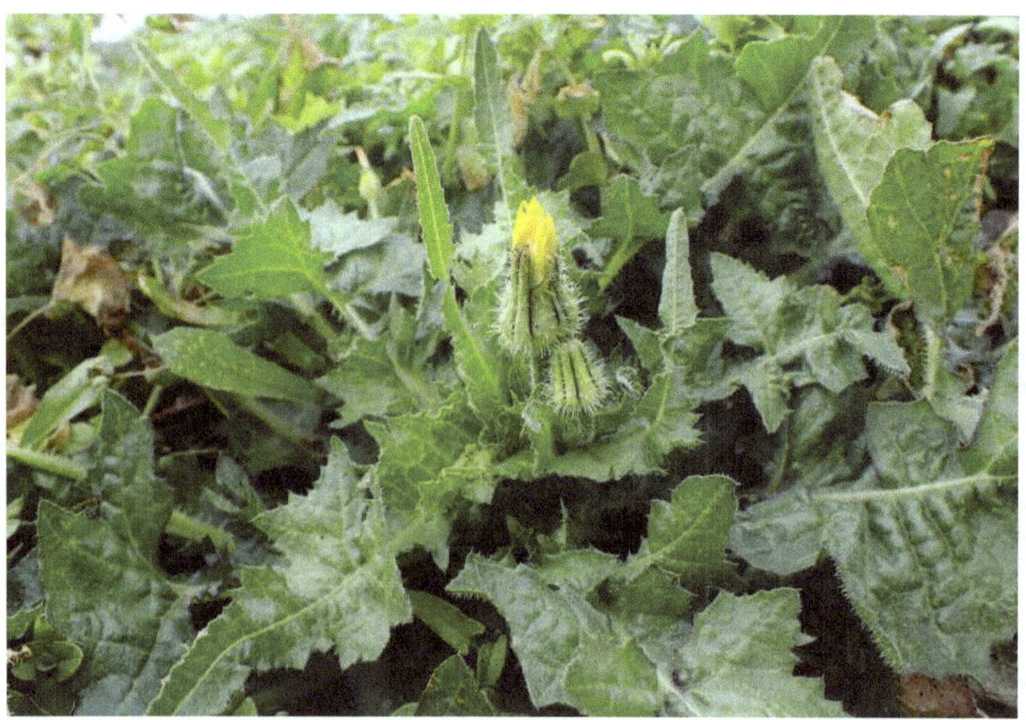

Photo by Krzysztof Ziarnek

Glystrída (Portulaca oleracea)

Glystrída—common purslane—is a perennial native plant distinguished by its sprawling, smooth, succulent, reddish stems that branch out and root at their nodes when in contact with soil. The plant's leaves grow in a rosette pattern, appearing spindle-shaped and fleshy with a silky texture and a rich green color. Small, bright yellow flowers develop at the tips of the stems.

The plant produces green capsules filled with tiny black seeds. Common purslane flourishes in cultivated lands, especially in irrigated vegetable gardens, during late spring. It has exceptional tolerance to drought and disease. The tender shoots are harvested from early summer until autumn.

This plant is rich in omega-3 fatty acids and offers nutrients like calcium, magnesium, iron, phosphorus, and copper, as well as vitamins A, C, B, and carotenoids. It has properties that can relieve pain, calm, reduce fever, lower blood pressure, and act as a diuretic. Additionally, it can benefit those with gallstones, provides antioxidants, and may protect against cancer, heart disease, and inflammation. However, it might reduce sexual desire.

Purslane is often consumed raw in salads, frequently paired with vinaigrette and added to summer tomato salads. It is also used in dishes with legumes, such as black beans, lentils, and chickpeas. People also include it in pickles and soups or cook it with meat or fish.

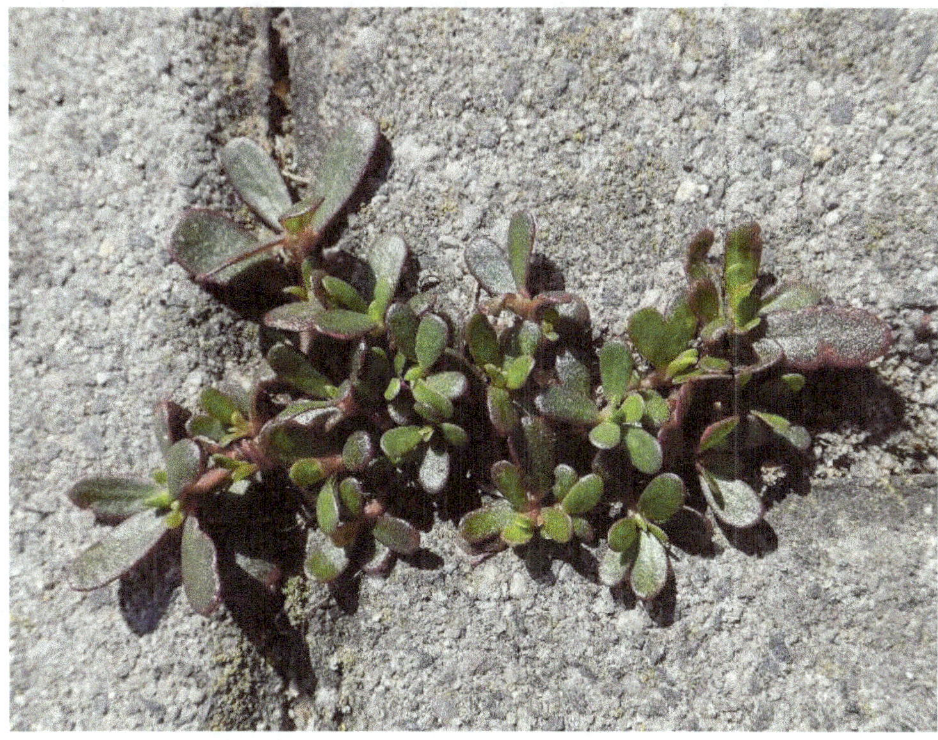

Photo by Salicyna

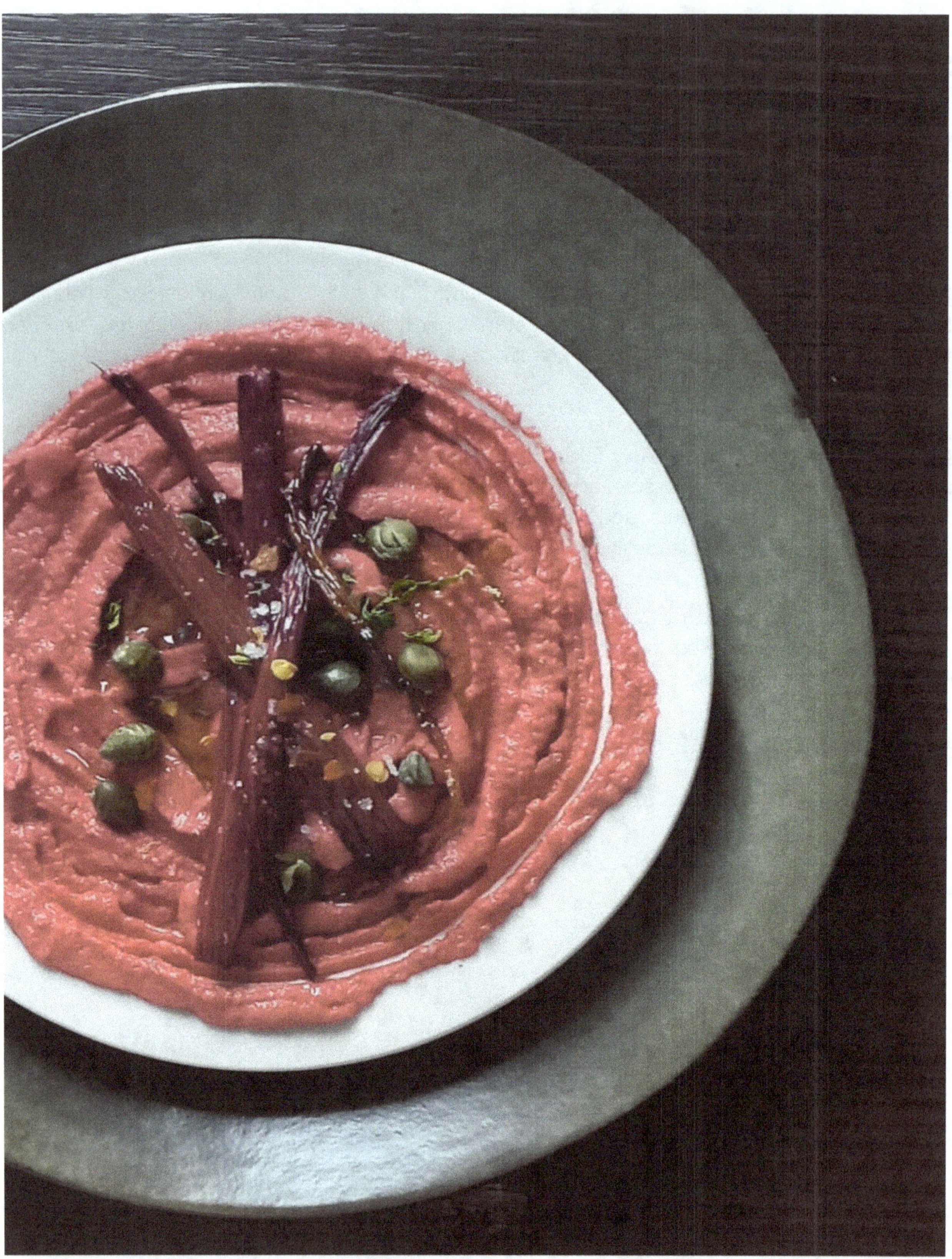

Cretan fava and beetroot topped with deep-fried beetroot, Cretan capers, and pepper flakes.

Kápari (Capparis spinosa)

Kápari—caper bush or Flinders rose—scientifically known as Capparis spinosa, is a perennial plant notable for its thorny features and horizontally growing young branches that can extend up to 1.5 meters. Its leaves are grey-green, thick, and smooth, arranged in an alternating pattern, and resemble an oval shape.

Small yellow spines appear near the base of its stems. The plant's flowers stand out for their size and long pedicels, producing a pleasant scent. These blossoms have four petals, which vary between white and violet, and include distinctive violet stamens with a stigma typically extending beyond the filaments.

Kápari flourishes in areas of low altitude where winters remain mild. It prefers rocky slopes, stony settings, olive groves, and both barren and cultivated fields, struggling in highly clayey or sandy soils.

Capers are known for their abundance of nutrients, including flavonoids, glycosides, polyprenols, beta-carotene, and vitamins C, E, and K. They also contain selenium, calcium, salt, magnesium, polyunsaturated fatty acids, and phytosterols.

Their tender stems, unopened buds, and fruits are frequently used to enhance the flavor of salads, dips, pickles, sauces, and various dishes. Often paired with seafood like salted cod or enjoyed with fava beans, capers are appreciated for their ability to stimulate appetite and deliver antioxidant, diuretic, and tonic benefits.

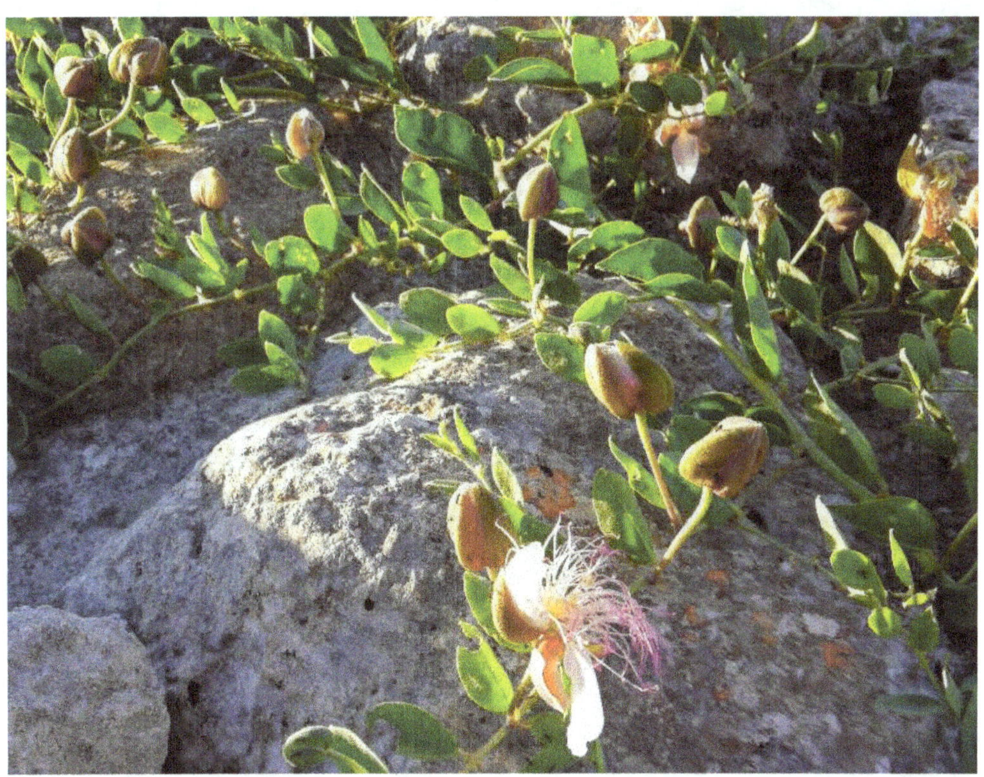

Kardamo (Capsella bursa pastoris)

Kardamo, or shepherd's purse, is an annual herb distinguished by a deep taproot. Its upright stem, covered with soft hairs, can reach up to 50 cm in height. The plant features basal leaves with serrated edges arranged in a rosette, while its upper leaves are sessile with two broad leaflets at their base and forming seed pods.

In its second year, it develops flowering stems that also grow to 50 cm. The small white flowers appear in clusters, bearing extended stalks, blooming year-round, producing green, triangular fruits with notches that resemble a heart. This plant adapts well to both poor and fertile soils and is commonly found along roads, gardens, and terraces.

Kardamo is a nutritional powerhouse with vitamins A, B, C, and K, as well as saponins, mustard oil, flavonoids, monoamines, resin, choline, acetylcholine, sitosterol, diosmin, calcium, iron, and potassium. Kardamo has medicinal properties that reduce inflammation, control bleeding, and fight bacterial infections. It also acts as a diuretic and astringent and shows anti-cancer potential, making it useful for treating cystitis and skin conditions.

However, it should not be used by those with thrombophlebitis. Its tender sprouts are eaten raw in salads, or its leaves are cooked with other greens in lemon-infused oil or added to soups.

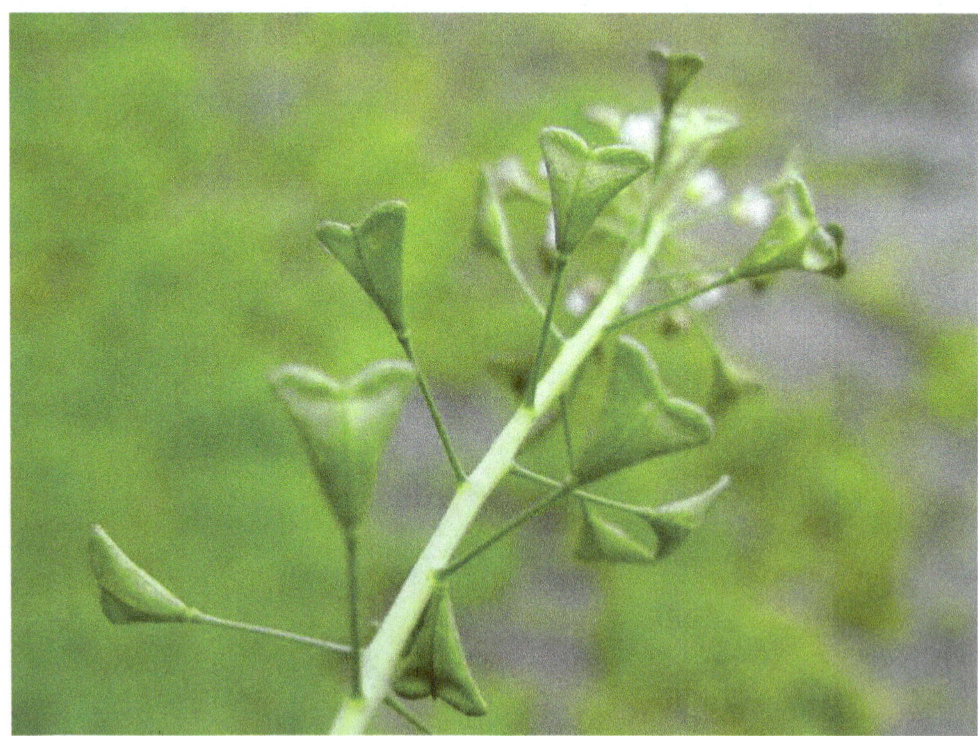

Photo by Harry Rose

Kavkalíthra (Tordylium apulum)

Kavkalithra—the Mediterranean hartwort or deer plant—known scientifically as Tordylium apulum, is a perennial herb native to the Mediterranean. The plant features an upright stem covered in tiny hairs, reaching up to 70 centimeters in height. It presents a compact root system. Leaves grow in pairs along the stems, boasting a feathery texture with fine hairs, often simple or lobed.

Small white flowers bloom on the upper stems in complex umbrella-shaped clusters during spring. As the fruit matures, it splits into two sections, each holding a single seed. The plant is riddled with oil-producing glands that secrete a distinctive essential oil.

Kavkalithra thrives in a mix of sandy, clay, and loamy soils, favoring sunny locations. It grows during winter and spring, typically in fields, meadows, and barren landscapes at low to medium elevations. The plant is high in calcium, potassium, and flavonoid compounds.

Medicinally, it is valued for its tonic effects on the nervous system, its diuretic properties, and its ability to assist with depression and indigestion.

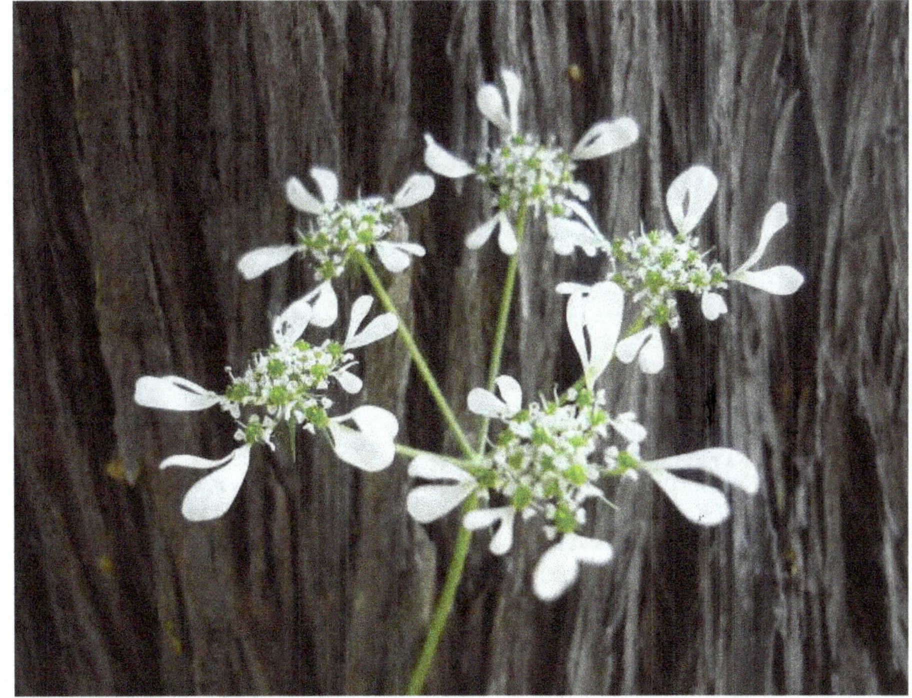

The leaves and young shoots are harvested in their tender phase from **winter to spring.**

Culinarily, it serves as a spice in small amounts within vegetable pies and other dishes, adding a unique taste and aroma.

It's often boiled or combined with various wild greens and used in meals like bean salads, fava bean meatballs, and fresh green salads.

Photo by Nick Savvopoulos

Klouvída (Chenopodium album)

Chenopodium album, commonly known as lamb's quarters, melde, or white goosefoot, is a nutrient-rich plant offering high calcium levels and vitamins A and C. Additionally, it contains small amounts of thiamin (B1), riboflavin (B2), niacin, iron, phosphorus, and potassium. Klouvída is noted for its anti-inflammatory, anti-rheumatic, and mild laxative properties, making it helpful for managing rheumatism.

This warm-season annual herb can grow up to 2.5 meters tall. Its stems often display ridges and may be tinted in shades of purple or red. The lower leaves are arranged alternately and vary in shape from rhombic to ovate, becoming more elliptic to linear as they ascend the stem. The leaves can reach up to 10 centimeters in length and have a distinct silvery-green hue on the underside due to a mealy bloom.

Flower clusters form in a branching pattern, with the larger clusters typically leafy. Flowers are bisexual or female, with perianth segments often fused halfway up, producing round, brown fruit, full of seeds. Klouvída adapts to various soil types but flourishes on fertile, heavy soils enriched with nitrogen or organic matter. It has spread as a weed across numerous crops worldwide, especially in cooler regions.

Leaves have traditionally been consumed as a green vegetable, while its seeds can be dried and ground into flour. Young plants are palatable to livestock.

The young shoots and leaves are often enjoyed boiled and added to salads with olive oil or pan-fried. They are also incorporated into pies and kalitsounias with other seasonal ingredients for enhanced flavor.

Kokkinogoúli (Crepis vesicaria)

Kokkinogoúli is a hardy perennial plant known in English as the beaked hawk's-beard. It features a strong taproot and an upright, branched stem covered in rough hairs, growing between 10 and 50 cm high. The lower leaves, connected directly to the stem, are elongated with pointed tips and can be either toothed or segmented into smaller parts. In contrast, the upper leaves are found on other plants, not rooted in the soil, exhibit a lanceolate form, and have lobed divisions.

The plant presents clusters of yellow flowers **from March to May**. Its fruit is a brown achene marked with distinct ridges. Kokkinogoúli thrives in cultivated lands and barren, rocky areas, such as olive groves and roadsides, at heights up to 600 meters.

It boasts significant nutritional benefits, being abundant in vitamins C and K, beta-carotene, flavonoids, and phenols, as well as minerals like magnesium, iron, phosphorus, sodium, potassium, manganese, and zinc. It also possesses notable antioxidant, anti-inflammatory, and antibacterial properties.

Before blooming—in February—the leaves and tender buds of Kokkinogoúli are edible, typically cooked with other vegetables, but in moderation due to their intense bitterness.

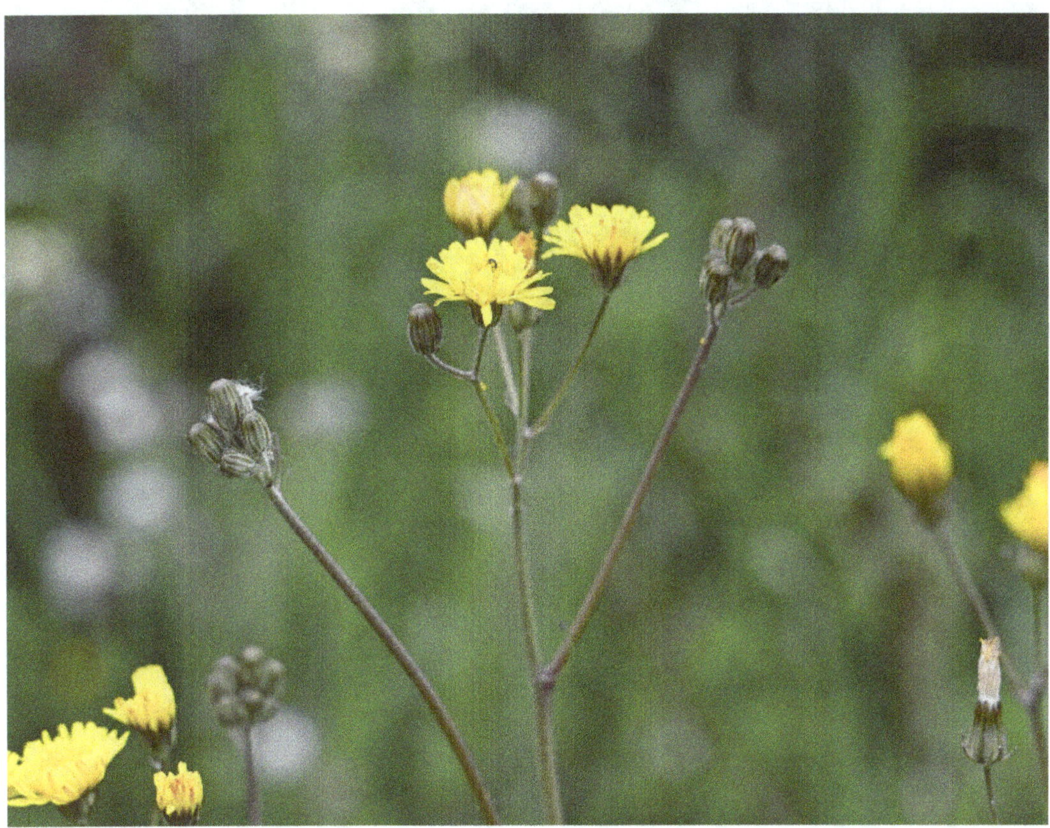

Photo by Krzysztof Ziarnek

Korakoúli (Scabiosa atropurpurea)

Korakoúli, known in English by various names like mourningbride, mournful widow, pincushion flower, or sweet scabious, is a perennial plant with a straight, T-shaped stem that can reach 80 cm in height and branch out. The plant features intricately arranged leaves; the lower ones appear rectangular and rhomboid, while the upper leaves are lobed and pinnate. Its floral arrangement showcases lilac and white flowers that bloom from June through September.

This plant thrives in unkempt fields, near farmland, within olive groves, by roadsides, in dry grasslands, scrubland, and open low-altitude areas. While not classified as a toxic plant, scabiosa is not commonly recognized among edible wild herbs. Nevertheless, it may possess medicinal properties, being sometimes categorized alongside medicinal plants. In Cretan folk tradition, Korakoúli is considered rich in antioxidants, which help lower blood sugar levels and shield the liver from damage.

From March to April, people consume boiled young shoots and immature basal leaves in early spring. Due to its strong, bitter taste, it is used sparingly.

Photo by Magnus Manske

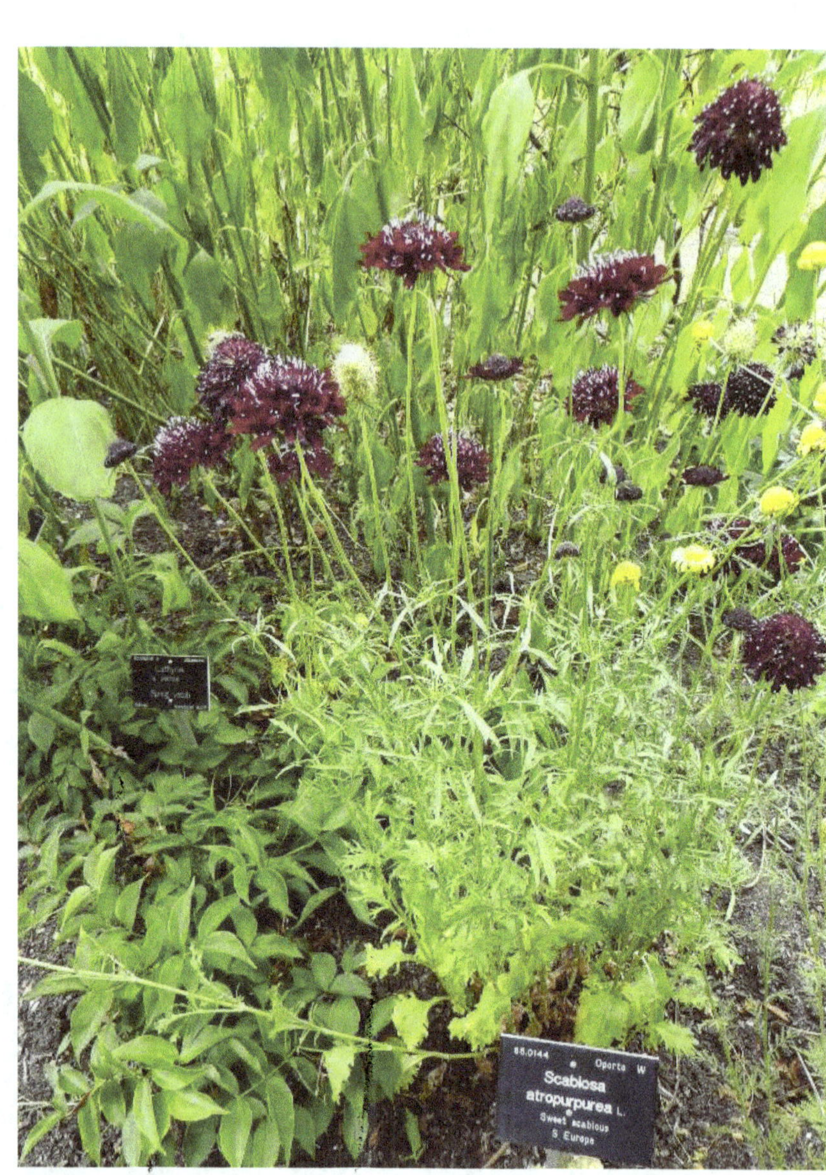

Koutsounáda (Papaver rhoeas)

Koutsounada, also known as the common poppy, corn poppy, field poppy, Flanders poppy, or red poppy, is a perennial herb. It features a strong main root and a hairy stem and exudes white to yellowish latex when broken. Its stems are straight, thin, and hollow.

The plant's leaves are moderately sized, long, and light green. Its large blossoms have two hairy sepals and four deep red petals with shiny black bases. These flowers bloom in spring, emerging from leaf joints on long, hairy stalks—the flowers droop before they open but stand tall afterwards. The plant produces an elongated capsule-shaped fruit containing 8 to 10 seeds.

This plant grows well in wild and farmed fields, grasslands, and sunny roadside areas. It favors rich, moist, and cohesive soil. Koutsounada contains alkaloids like papaverine and rhoeadine, along with meconic acid, tannin, iron, manganese, potassium, calcium, and various acids. The poppy has calming, moisturizing, cough-suppressing, sedative, and mildly sweat-inducing qualities.

Cretans eat the young stems and leaves by cooking them with other greens in stews. They're also added to vegetable soups and pies. The fragrant seeds sometimes replace sesame in baked goods and sweets.

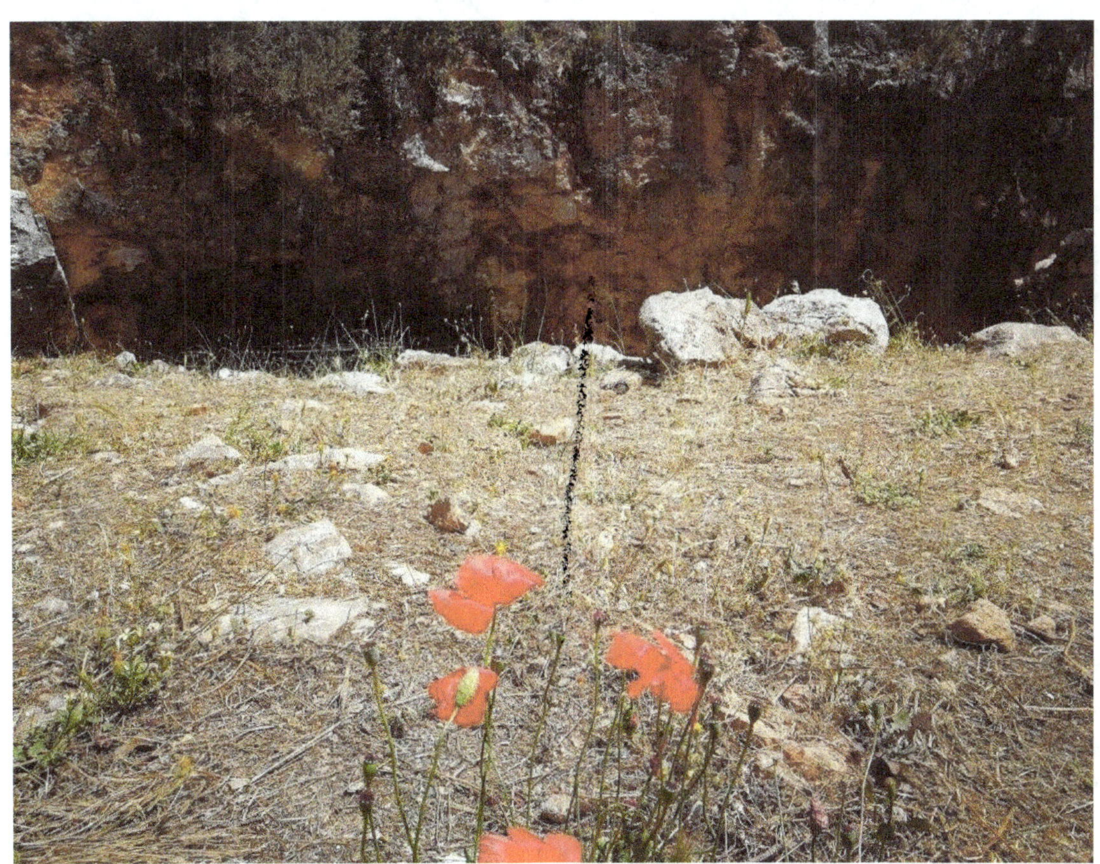

Krítamos (Crithmum maritimum)

Krítamos—Crithmum maritimum—or, In English, rock samphire, sea fennel, or samphire, is a low-growing perennial grass. Its straight shoots can branch out and display stripes, reaching heights of up to 60 centimeters with a blue-green tint. The plant's base is woody, smooth, and fleshy, featuring creeping roots. Its elongated, succulent leaves have a silk-like texture and deep green color, emerging from swollen nodes. The plant is characterized by an inflorescence called an umbel, with small, greenish-white flowers. Its fruit is oval and spongy.

This plant thrives in coastal and rocky settings, such as rock crevices and sandy beaches, favoring well-drained soils with neutral pH. Krítamos is well-suited to warm climates and requires minimal soil moisture, showing a high resistance to salt. Rich in trace minerals and talc salts, including iodine and vitamins E, O, and K, Krítamos is an excellent source of antioxidants and omega-3 fatty acids.

The leaves and young shoots are harvested before flowering and used in salads like country, tomato, or potato salads, adding flavor when drizzled with olive oil. They complement drinks like tsikoudia, ouzo, or tsipouro and pair well with fish and meat dishes. The branches and petals can be sautéed for omelets.

Apart from culinary uses, Krítamos offers moderate antioxidant benefits, aids detoxification, purifies blood, and supports liver health. It acts as a diuretic and boosts appetite.

The essential oil of Krítamos is known for its aphrodisiac properties.

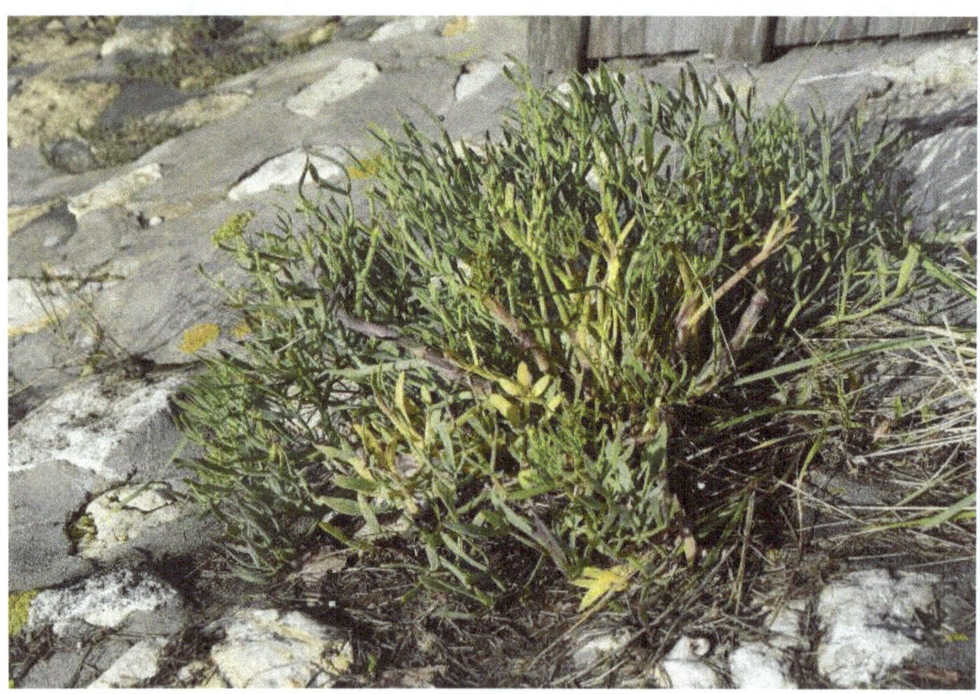

Lagoudóchorto (Prasium majus)

Lagoudóchorto—scientifically Prasium majus and in English white hedge-nettle—is a perennial shrub between 70 and 100 cm tall. Its stem is upright and smooth, branching irregularly. The leaves are opposite, short-stemmed, either oval or heart-shaped with serrated edges, and exhibit a green hue. During its blooming period from April to May, this plant displays striking white-pink flowers growing in pairs from the axils. These flowers feature bell-shaped calyxes with a hairy interior.

The plant prospers in meadows, scrublands, infertile fields, uncultivated slopes, and rocky limestone areas, thriving at elevations up to 600 meters. It is notable for its high concentrations of vitamins A, C, and K, as well as lutein, beta-carotene, and polyphenols.

Lagoudóchorto is valued for its aromatic stems and leaves, often used in cooking. Common preparations include frying and incorporation into dishes like vegetable pies, egg sfugato, and stews with cuttlefish and snails.

Beyond its culinary uses, this plant is acknowledged for its digestive benefits. It aids in the healing of stomach and duodenal ulcers and helps manage gastric acid secretion. When taken as a beverage, it may help reduce fever and energize the body.

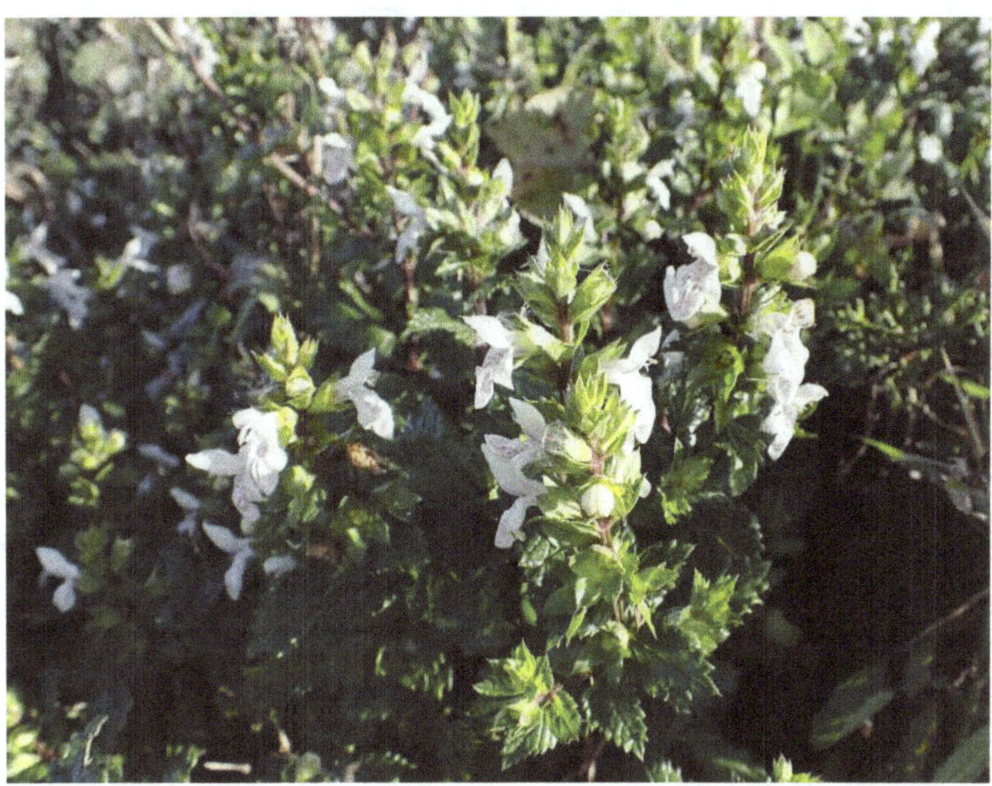

Lápatho (Rumex acetosa)

Lápatho—common sorrel or garden sorrel—is a biennial plant. It can grow between 10 to 50 centimeters tall, and its flowering stem might extend up to 100 centimeters. Lápatho's leaves are either lance-shaped or heart-shaped near the base and are attached to long stalks. The plant produces small, dioecious flowers arranged in dense, reddish spikes. These flowers typically bloom from April to May.

Lápatho thrives in damp soils that are either acidic, neutral, or alkaline, regardless of sunlight exposure. The leaves are rich in vitamins A and E, iron, calcium, phosphorus, antioxidants, and flavonoids, but due to high oxalate levels, they should be consumed in moderation.

Lápatho contains phytoestrogens, which have diuretic, fever-reducing, and bile-regulating properties. It also has anti-inflammatory effects. The plant's high quercetin content helps prevent cardiovascular diseases.

The primary culinary use of Lápatho leaves is in vegetable pies, but they also serve as wraps for dolmades. They can be cooked alone or paired with meat and are often mashed for soups.

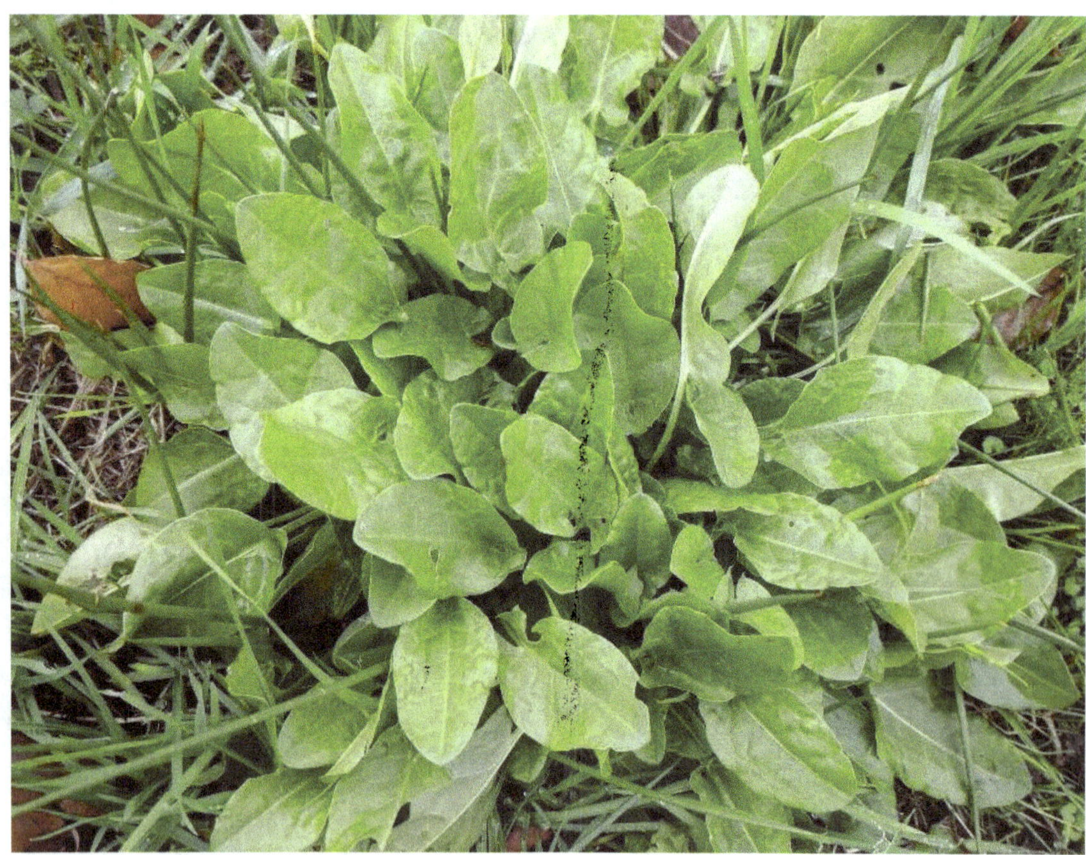

Photo by Michel Langeveld

Leivadítis (Pimpinella peregrina)

Leivaditis—southern burnet saxifrage (Pimpinella peregrina or Anisum italicum)—is a biennial herb characterized by a tall, striped stem that can grow up to 1 meter high. Its structure features branches and a covering of leaves, where the lower ones are arranged in a pinnate fashion with heart-shaped, toothed leaflets. In contrast, the middle leaves are wedge-shaped with teeth, and the upper leaves are slender and linear.

The flowers are white, and the fruit displays a covering of erect hairs—this plant blooms in April and May. Leivadítis thrives in rocky and sloped terrains located in lowland and semi-mountainous areas. It is also commonly seen in olive groves, by roadsides, and along the edges of streams and rivers.

It is available for consumption **from January to March**, offering a pleasing sweetness and taste. Its leaves and tender shoots are typically eaten smoked, incorporated into pies, or included in kalitsounia, often mixed with other greens for added flavor.

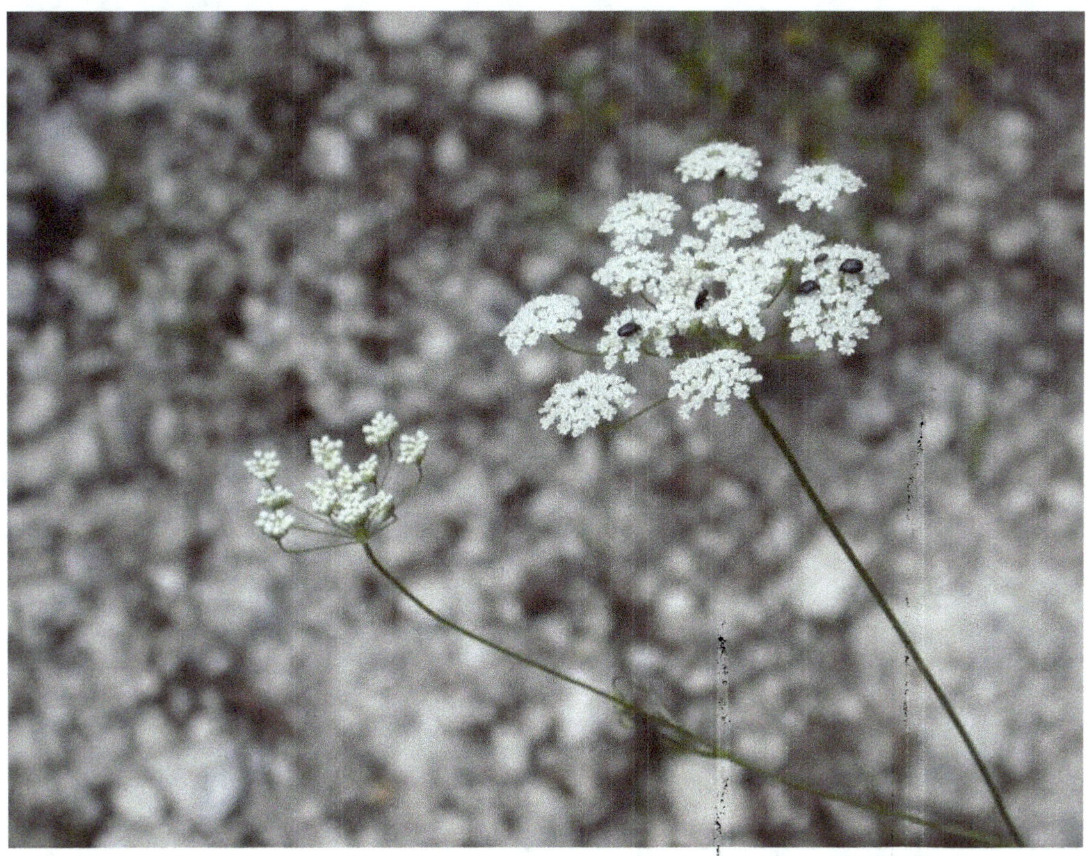

Photo by Gideon Pisanty

Mantilída (Glebionis coronaria)

Mantilída, scientifically known as Glebionis coronaria (formerly Chrysanthemum coronarium), is an annual plant that can reach heights up to 1.20 meters. It has several English names, including garland chrysanthemum, chrysanthemum greens, edible chrysanthemum, crowndaisy chrysanthemum, chop suey greens, crown daisy, and Japanese greens.

With a svelte stem and multiple branches, it showcases numerous bipinnate leaves. The flower heads measure around 5 to 6 cm across, displaying blooms that are typically yellow or white with a yellow center, and are hermaphroditic.

This plant prefers habitats like barren fields, roadside areas, ditches, and cultivated lands in hilly and semi-hilly regions. It thrives in well-drained soils that maintain adequate moisture levels. Nutritionally, this plant contains 27.7% protein, 4.6% fat, 50.8% carbohydrates, 13.8% fiber, and essential minerals such as calcium, phosphorus, iron, magnesium, sodium, potassium, and zinc. It's also rich in vitamins A, B1, B2, niacin, and C, along with essential amino acids.

Mantilída is beneficial in managing cardiovascular conditions and has both expectorant and tartaric effects.

The tender shoots and stems of the Mantilída are edible and can be enjoyed raw in salads or boiled with other greens. Once stripped of their leaves, the young shoots can be eaten raw with vinegar or cooked briefly with the leaves or flowers and added to salads.

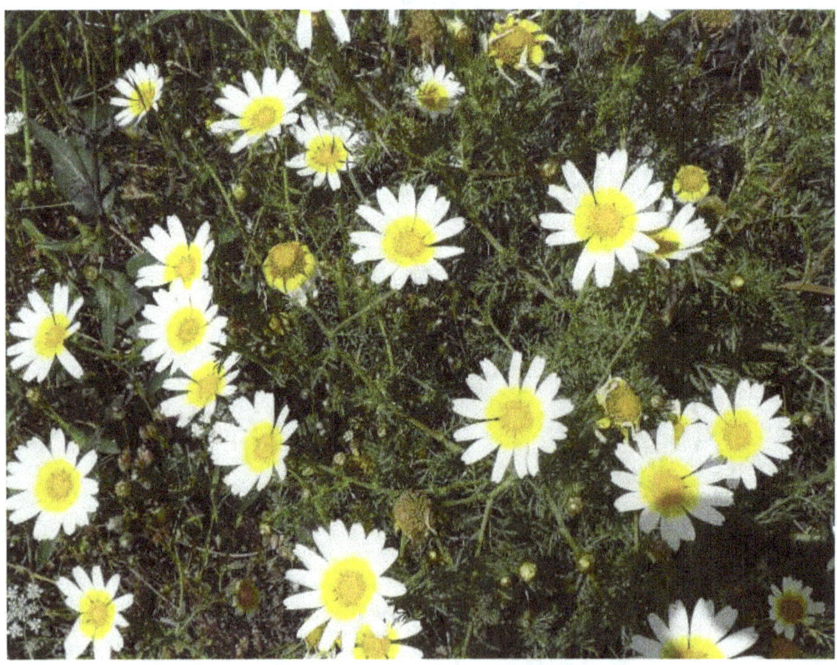

Máratho (Foeniculum vulgare)

Máratho, in English fennel, is a perennial plant with a tall, sturdy, and smooth-striped stem with numerous branches, reaching heights up to two meters. The root is notable for its robust and fleshy nature, from which the stem arises. The leaves are deep green, with long stalks and a compound, pinnate form. Fennel produces small yellow flowers arranged in umbrella-like clusters, typically blooming between June and August.

The plant yields small, oval fruits with striped markings, appearing in a yellowish or brown shade, usually harvested from August to September.

Fennel prefers thriving in uncultivated spaces along waterways, roadsides, and terraced slopes. It favors well-drained, sunny soils rich in nutrients, with a pH ranging from 5.5 to 6.5. Known for its high content of volatile oils such as estragole, anethole, and fenchone, fennel is also rich in vitamins A, C, E, K, and B6. It includes fatty acids, flavonoids, amino acids like histidine and arginine, and minerals such as calcium, potassium, phosphorus, and magnesium.

Fennel boasts several health benefits. It acts as a diuretic, boosts appetite, serves as a tonic, regulates menstrual cycles, aids in lactation, helps expel fatty compounds, and soothes conditions like bronchitis and cough.

Every part of the fennel plant—roots, stems, leaves, and seeds—can be consumed. It is a staple in many fasting dishes, such as artichokes, dolmades, octopus, cuttlefish, snails, fried greens, and black-eyed beans. It's a main ingredient in marathopitas, wild greens, pies, and horta kalitsuna. Fennel adds flavor to olives and pickles. Its seeds find use both as a culinary spice and a medicinal herb.

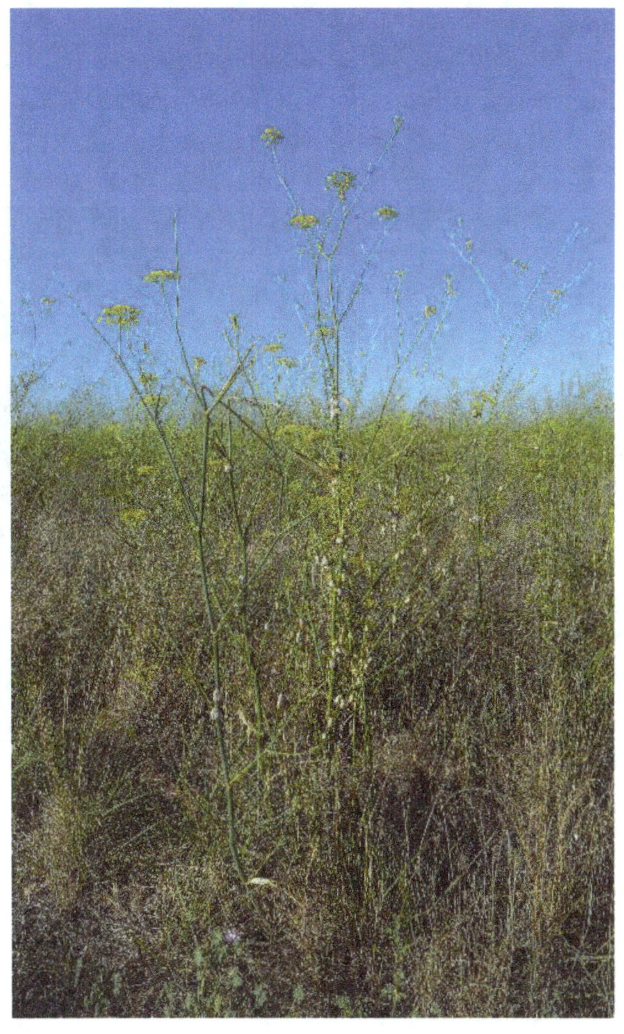

Melissóchorto (Melissa officinalis)

Melissóchorto—lemon balm—is a hardy perennial plant with an upright growth habit and can reach up to 90 centimeters in height. Its roots are cylindrical, robust, and fibrous. The leaves are oval with a light coating of hairs, serrated edges, and a blunt or heart-shaped base. They have a light green hue and exude a faint citrusy scent. During summer, small white flowers that are rich in nectar appear.

This plant thrives in wooded and bushy areas, especially in southern-facing hilly regions near stream edges. It prefers well-drained soils that are moderately nutrient-rich and medium in texture. Crete's regional climate experiences a dry season from June to October, yet lemon balm thrives here, too, mainly in gorges, and the island boasts over 400 such natural formations.

Lemon balm is rich in polyphenols, tannins, rosmarinic acid, flavonoids, and essential oils like citral, citronellal, linalool, and geraniol. The plant's leaves are collected twice a year. In culinary contexts, honeysuckle leaves enhance the aroma and taste of dishes, notably fish recipes. They are often cooked in a method known as yahni or served as a flavorful side dish with pork or lamb in a dish called

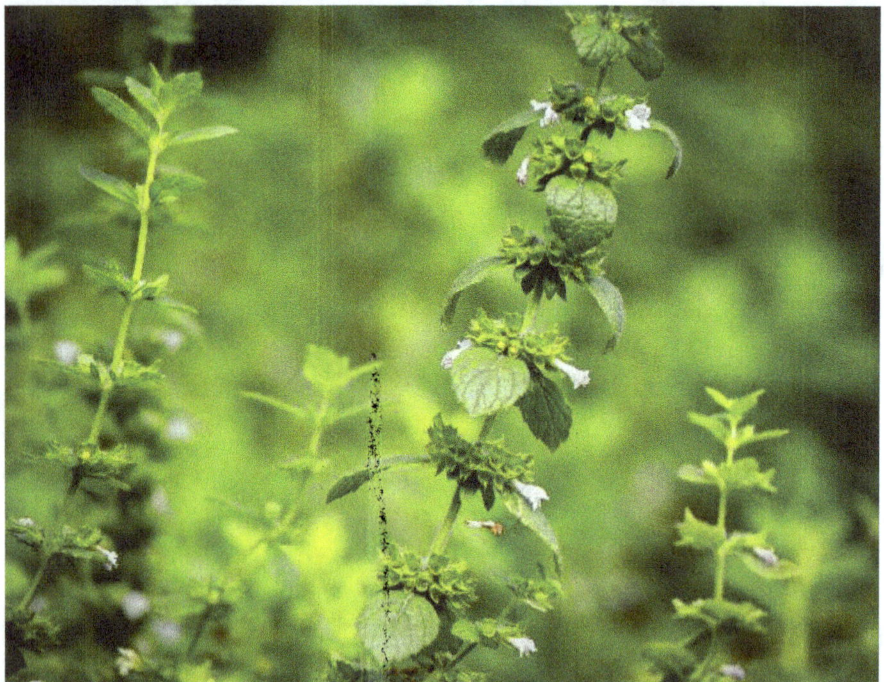

tsoukali. Additionally, the leaves can be enjoyed raw in salads, offering a refreshing taste.

They are also used to flavor alcoholic beverages, including beer, liqueurs, and wines.

Melissóchorto has antispasmodic, anti-inflammatory, and antibacterial properties. It supports heart function and blood circulation, aiding in the fight against viral infections and cold sores. Furthermore, it can help reduce anxiety and alleviate gastrointestinal distress. Studies indicate its potential in easing symptoms for those with Alzheimer's disease.

Molócha (Malva sylvestris)

Molócha - common mallow - is a perennial herbaceous plant characterized by an upright stem with several branches, capable of attaining a height of up to 150 cm. The leaves are palm-shaped with rounded edges, split into five lobes. Each lobe has a long and slender stem. The flower emerges from the stalk and often displays a pink hue with purple rays. However, its appearance may differ depending on the locality. It is composed of five petals and an anther. The fruit has a flat shape and has a large number of segments.

This plant has a wide distribution and thrives in many habitats, such as roadsides, fallow and cultivated fields, gardens, and residential areas, without specific environmental demands. Molócha is composed of flavonoids, glycine, and minor quantities of vitamins A, B1, B2, and C. It also includes traces of tannin, while its blossoms are abundant in anthocyanosides.

Molócha leaves provide soothing properties that alleviate irritation of the mucous membranes. They are recommended for individuals suffering from bronchitis, dry coughs, and sore throats. They are also used to treat ailments affecting the digestive and urinary systems, such as colic, cystitis, and gastritis. Furthermore, they aid in managing intestinal illnesses and assist in addressing kidney and liver issues.

The plant is consumed in its whole, including the leaves and vulnerable shoots, before blooming. The leaves may boiled or sautéed and are commonly used in salads, pies, and soups. However, their slimy texture may not appeal to everyone. Due to their high nitrate content, it is recommended to consume them in moderation.

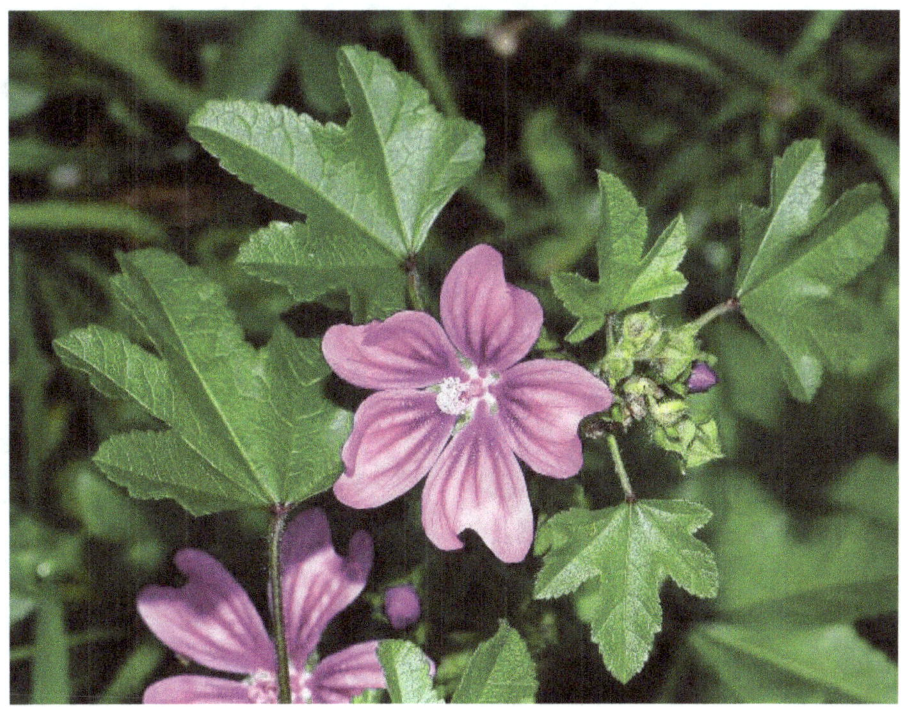

Pentaneuro (Plantago major)

Pentaneuro—broadleaf plantain, white man's footprint, waybread, or greater plantain—has a biennial growth cycle and reaches between 15 and 30 centimeters in height. It is identifiable by its large, broad, dark green leaves formed in an oval-elliptical shape, arranged in a rosette at the base. From this base, a tall stalk arises, supporting cylindrical spikes populated with numerous small greenish flowers.

This resilient plant thrives independently in diverse settings, such as abandoned fields, urban areas, and along roadsides. Pentaneuro is rich in carotene, vitamins C and K, glycosides, tannins, organic acids, mucilage, saponins, enzymes, and alkaloids.

Pentaneuro offers diuretic, antibacterial, and wound-healing properties. It helps lower blood lipid levels, including triglycerides, cholesterol, and lipoproteins while boosting good cholesterol, which is beneficial in preventing heart disease.

After removing the stems, the young leaves are edible and can be added to salads with other vegetables, included in soups, mixed into omelets, or cooked alongside various wild and cultivated greens.

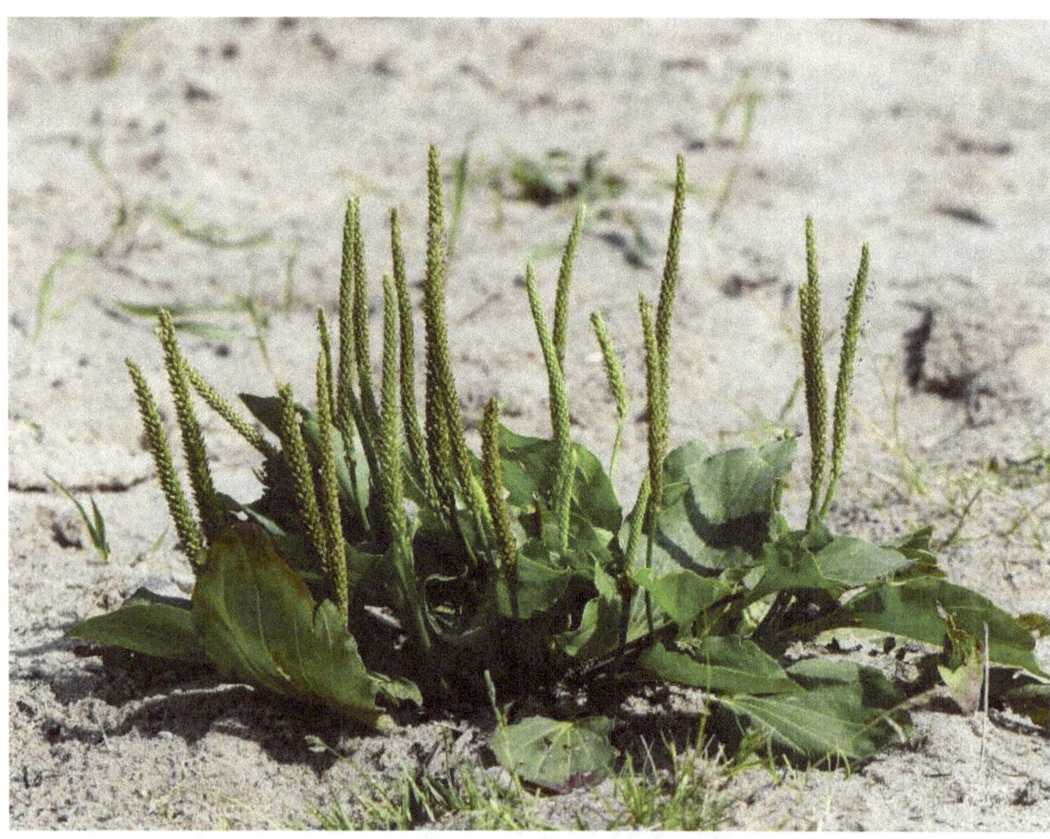

Image by Krzysztof Ziarnek

Perdikoúli (Anagallis arvensis)

Perdikoúli, also known as scarlet pimpernel, red pimpernel, red chickweed, poor man's barometer, poor man's weather-glass, shepherd's weather glass, or shepherd's clock, is a small perennial plant. It remains low to the ground, growing only 1 to 10 cm in height.

The plant's shoots appear rectangular when viewed from the side. Its small leaves are paired, lacking stems, and are elliptical with distinct secretory features. These tiny flowers grow from where the leaves meet and bloom during April and May.

It thrives in low-altitude areas, finding suitable habitats in abandoned and cultivated fields, along roadsides, and on dirt paths. It prefers light, moist soils and avoids direct sunlight. Perdikoúli contains potassium nitrate, tannins, saponins, glycosides, essential oil, and curcuvitacins.

Although mildly toxic, with poisonous seeds and leaf contact potentially causing skin irritation, young leaves are edible in small amounts, raw or cooked, and often added to salads for their bitter taste. Known for its diuretic properties, Perdikoúli is also a mild astringent. It provides a refreshing effect and helps treat genitourinary system disorders.

Photo by Hans Hillewaert

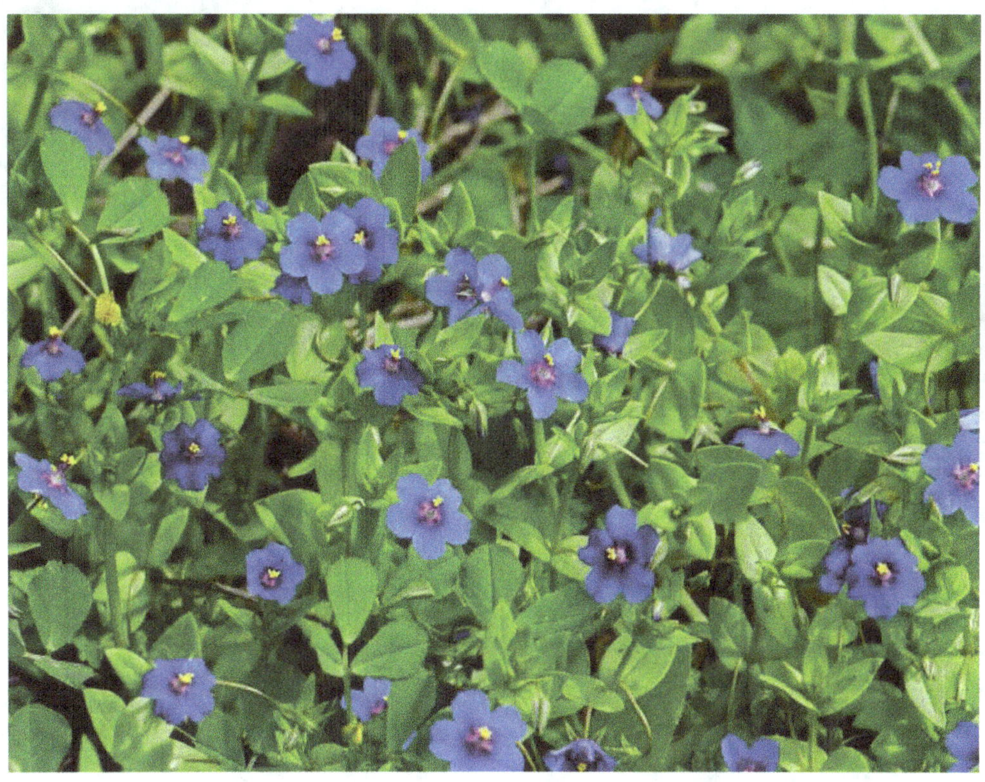

Petrómaroulo (Lactuca serriola)

Petrómaroulo—also known as prickly lettuce, compass plant, or scarole—is a biennial plant notable for its tiny, three-part leaves with an upright stem that can reach a height of 80 cm. Its fleshy and serrated leaves form a rosette pattern at the base.

The stem is hair-covered, featuring a central vein with rigid, thorny hairs and lacks stalks. The upper sides of the leaves are dark green and glossy, while the undersides are lighter. Both its shoots and leaves release a milky sap.

The plant produces clusters of pale yellow flowers consisting of numerous tongue-shaped florets. It bears fruits filled with many small, elongated seeds.

It thrives in fallow lands, cultivated fields, and along roadsides, favoring infertile, rocky, and dry soils.

Petrómaroulo is rich in nutrients such as vitamins A, B1, B2, C, and iron and contains flavonoids, lactones, coumarins, and mannitol. It has sedative effects that promote restful sleep and help reduce anxiety and restlessness. It also possesses diuretic and tartaric qualities. Its bitterness increases as it matures and

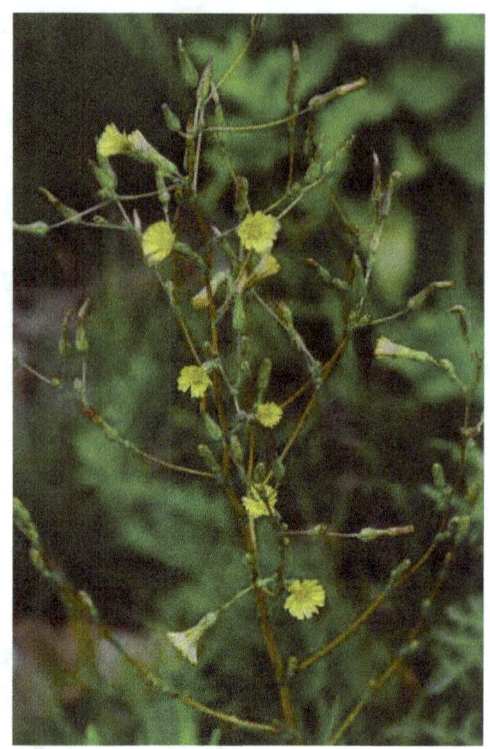

blooms.

The young leaves and stems are typically boiled briefly and used in salads and other leafy greens.

Photo by Krzysztof Ziarnek

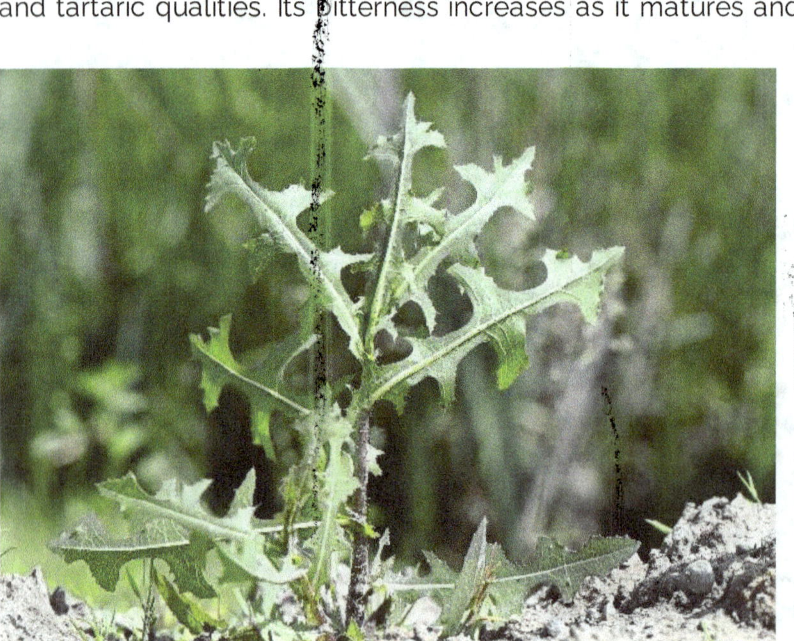

Petrofiliá (Petromarula pinnata)

Petromarula pinnata, known as Petrofiliá, is a perennial herb that thrives in clusters. It grows with leaves spreading near the ground and tall, smooth stems rising above. The basal leaves are long, attached by stalks, and arranged in a pattern resembling feathers. Their tops are either spearhead-shaped or heart-shaped, while the sides curve like sickles, edged with small teeth. The flowers are arranged in circular formations, clustered along a shared stem.

Petromarula pinnata is a **unique species native to Crete** in the Mediterranean region. The name "Petromarula" comes from the Greek, meaning "rock lettuce," a nod to its traditional use in salads.

Flowering is observed between April and June. This plant favors shaded and moist environments, often found on limestone rocks, rocky slopes, mountains, and rugged soils and terraces, reaching elevations up to 1200 meters.

The leaves are primarily consumed, while the tender shoots are also prized. They are used in various ways, such as smoking or in culinary dishes like pies and kalitsounia, particularly in conjunction with other seasonal greens available **from March to April.**

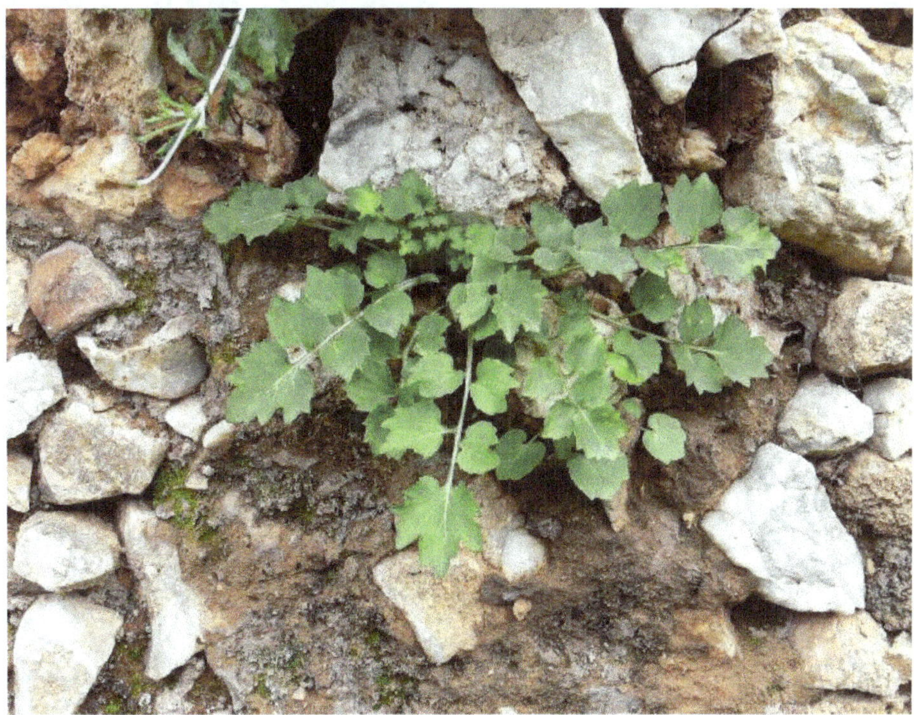

Photo by Wolfgang Sauber

Pigounítis (Tragopogon sinuatus)

Pigounítis, or Tragopogon sinuatus, is a biennial weed with a sturdy taproot and an upright stem reaching heights up to 60 cm. Its leaves exhibit a light green, linear-lanceolate shape with a noticeable central groove, becoming wider at the base and appearing sheathed. The plant's blooms are composed of a head featuring tongue-shaped flowers in pink or violet, typically appearing **from April to May**.

The fruit forms a spindle-like achene with minute scales arranged in rows. The plant contains a somewhat bitter, milky sap. Pigounítis flourishes in meadows, scrublands, roadsides, and other dry regions, often found at altitudes as high as 800 meters.

It is rich in various nutrients—vitamins C, K1, α-tocopherol, β-carotene, flavonoids, phenols, lutein, potassium, sodium, calcium, magnesium, iron, zinc, and phosphorus. Pigounítis has diuretic and laxative effects, which help reduce high blood pressure. Additionally, it finds use in treating arthritis, rheumatism, and various skin conditions.

The tender young shoots and leaves are edible, and the plant's succulent roots are traditionally cooked with leafy greens. It offers a sweet, savory flavor, enhancing a range of dishes when sautéed with other seasonal herbs.

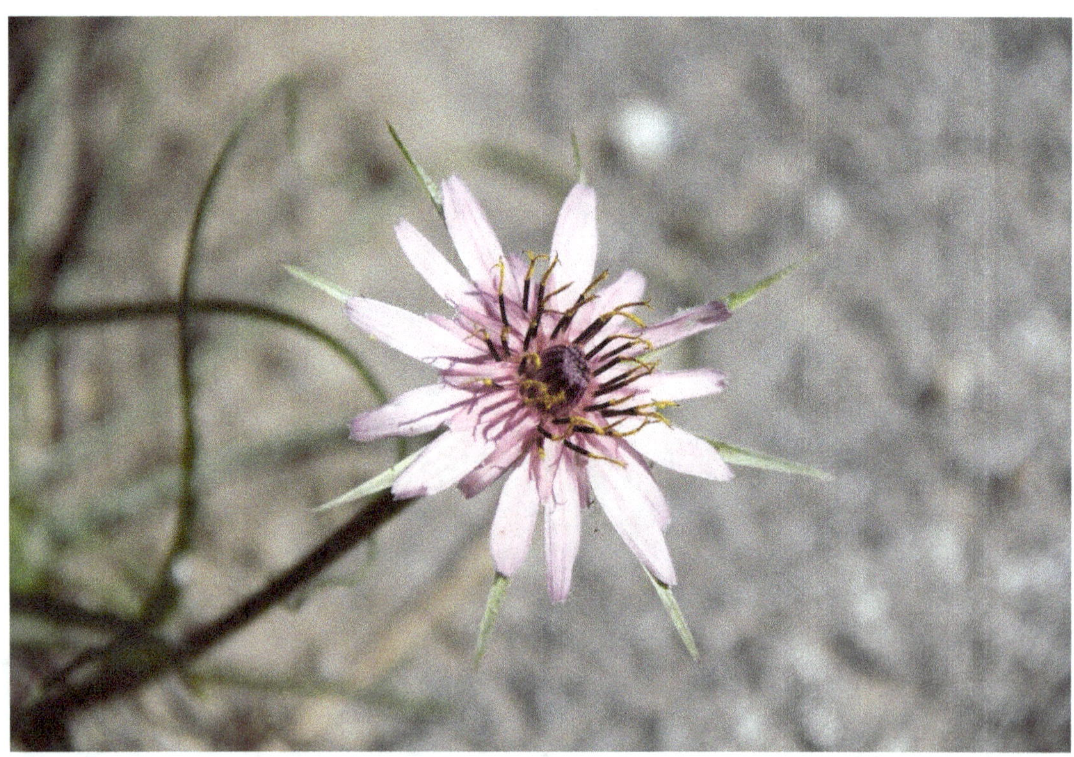

Pikróvrouva (Hirschfeldia incana)

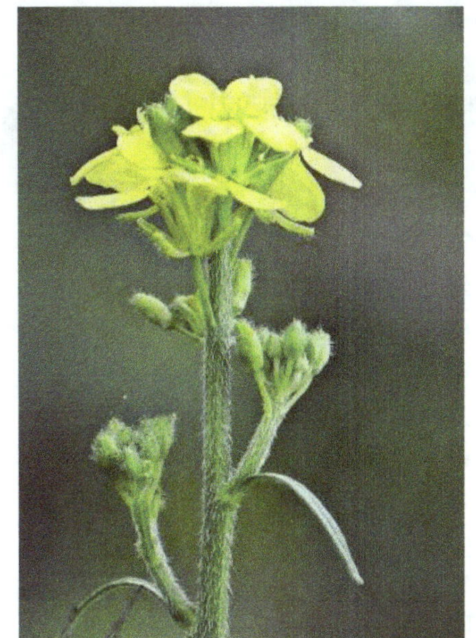

Pikróvrouva — also known as shortpod mustard, buchanweed, hoary mustard, and Mediterranean mustard — is a perennial herb that grows upright on a solitary stem with few branches and limited foliage, reaching up to 1 meter high. Its basal leaves form a dense cluster and are intricately arranged, with pinnate divisions into five lobes, the largest of which has toothed edges and a thin membrane along the teeth. The plant's flowers are small and yellow, gathered in clusters, while its fruit is short, horn-shaped, cylindrical, and slightly grooved.

Pikróvrouva flourishes in areas with low to moderate elevation, such as vineyards, orchards, field borders, riverbeds, streams, and roadsides.

It is packed with antioxidants, including vitamin C, beta-carotene, lutein, and zeaxanthin, and is a good source of B vitamins, folate, and vitamin K. This plant boasts digestive, cleansing, detoxifying, tonic, and diuretic properties that benefit the heart and circulatory system.

Young sprouts are boiled and added to salads with olive oil, and the inflorescences are often fried with eggs.

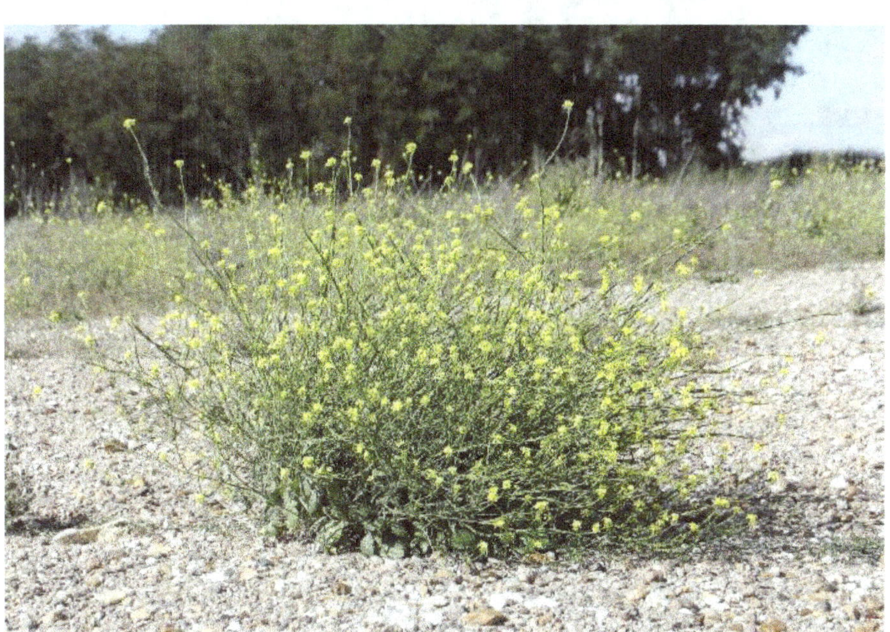

Pikrorádiko (Taraxacum officinale)

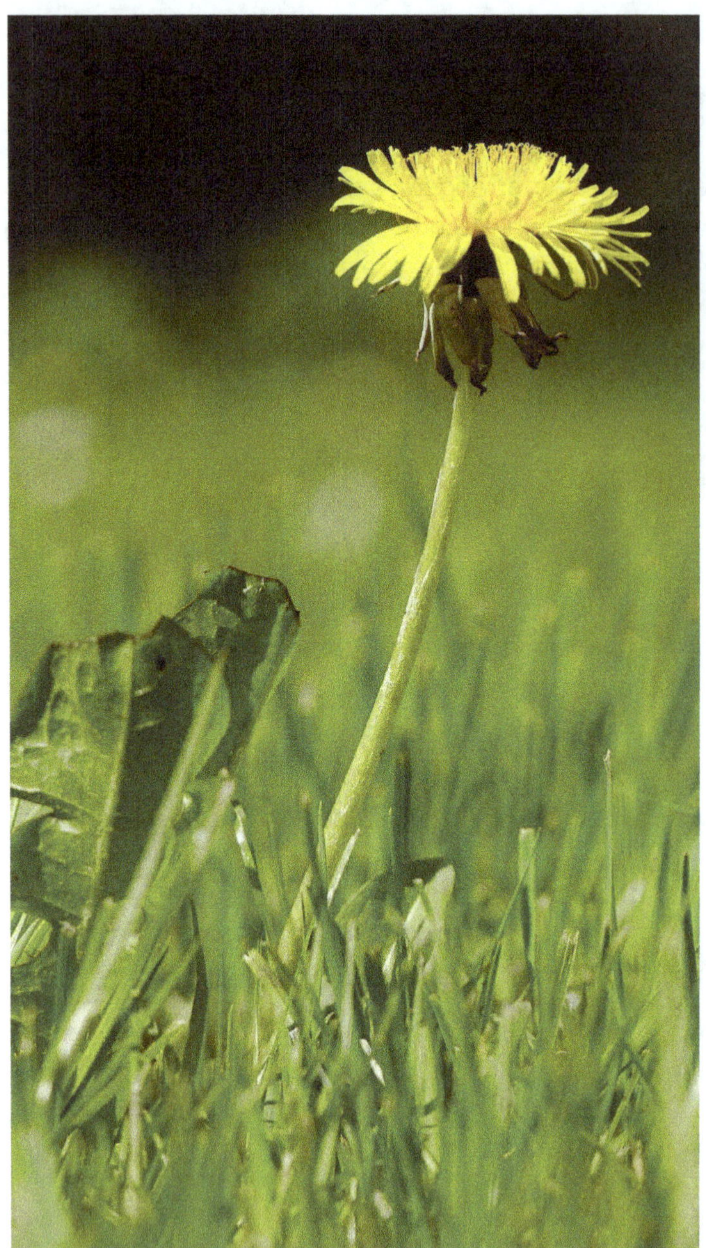

Pikrorádiko—or dandelion (Taraxacum officinale)—is a small plant with a compact arrangement of leaves, typically ranging from a single leaf up to ten.

These leaves extend outward in a circle from the base, resembling a feathered design. Some sections of the leaves exhibit a distinct triangular form with sharp points, tapering to become longer and narrower toward the tip.

The plant culminates in a flower head composed of numerous golden florets that blossom outward, starting from the center. It blooms during the spring and produces fruit known as achene.

It flourishes in both dry and moist soils, often in areas laden with gravel or stones, such as neglected fields, alongside roads, riverbanks, and similar spots.

It is rich in essential nutrients like potassium, vitamins A and C, iron, magnesium, and calcium. Furthermore, it contains flavonoids, terpenoids, sterols, and carotenoids, including lutein, violaxanthin, and polysaccharides.

Possessing both diuretic and tonic qualities, its decoction can be used to treat chronic conditions such as dermatitis, arthritis, mental fatigue, and persistent eczema.

It helps alleviate constipation and acts as an effective liver tonic, facilitating the removal of toxins while promoting liver health. In addition, it aids in reducing cholesterol and regulating blood sugar levels.

Dandelion is often consumed after boiling with other wild greens, making it a popular ingredient in salads, vegetable pies, and kalitsounias.

Pirounáki (Erodium cicutarium)

Pirounáki—also known as stork's bill, redstem filaree, redstem stork's bill, or pinweed—features astringent, hemostatic, and antioxidant properties. It also exhibits a strong estrogenic and anti-inflammatory effect. This perennial herbaceous plant showcases a forked structure with deeply divided stems that arise from its base. It can grow upright or spread along the ground, reaching between 10 and 40 centimeters in height, with a hairy texture.

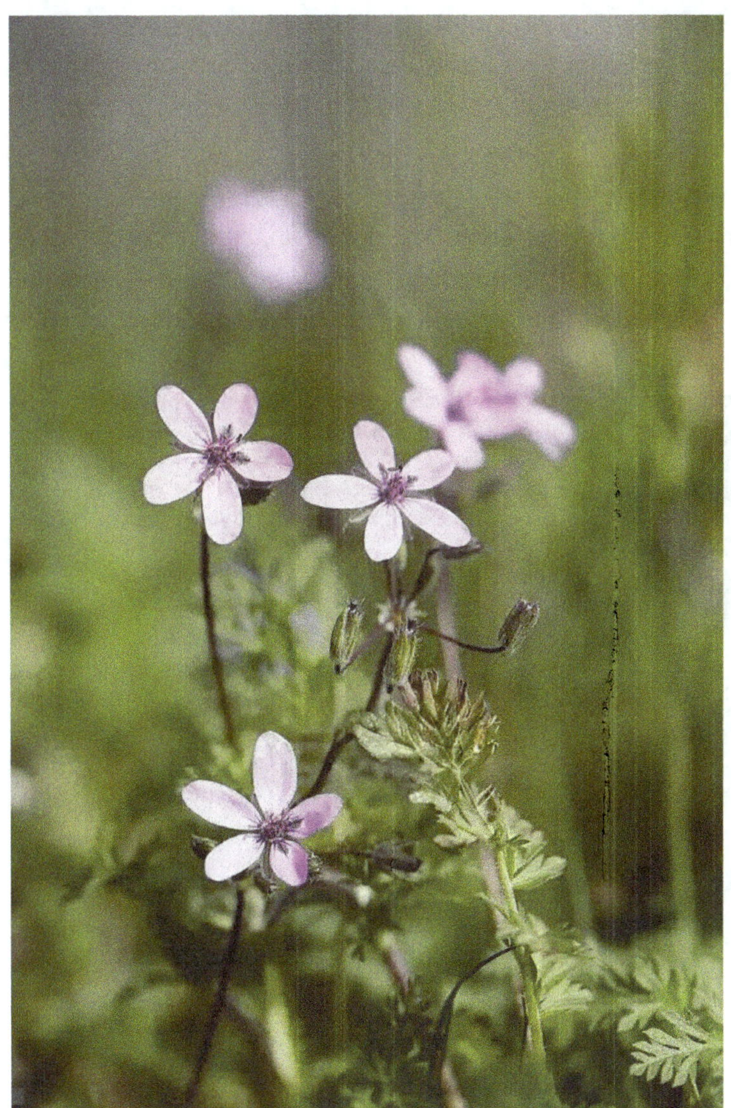

The leaves grow alternately and are green, oblong, with serrated edges. They possess a downy surface and have small wings at the base.

Flowers sprout in clusters from the leaf axils, presenting 2 to 8 small petals in pink, purple, or white hues.

Each flower has five petals and blooms from March to June. Its fruit is notable for its long beak, extending up to 2 centimeters, and contains a spiral-shaped seed with a tough fiber at its tip. Pirounáki thrives in moist soils at elevations from 100 to 1,600 meters.

It commonly appears in pastures, roadsides, meadows, and well-lit cultivated fields.

Composed of essential oils with elements like fatty acids, hexadecanoic acid, psyllium, ketones, tetracosane, minerals, and vitamin K, Pirounáki leaves can be an ingredient in omelets and horta pies.

Radíki (Cichorium intybus)

Radíki—the common chicory—is a perennial weed with a tall, upright, and multi-branched stem that can reach up to one meter in height. The plant displays a long, pointed base, and its stem ranges from smooth to slightly hairy. Its asymmetrical, broad, lance-shaped leaves grow directly from the stem, with the lower leaves often divided into leaflets. Its flowers form rounded clusters at the leaf axils, featuring both male and female parts and a striking blue color.

The flowers open early in the day, blooming **from July through October.** The plant produces a type of achene as fruit, containing numerous elongated seeds. Radíki grows well on rocky, dry slopes, along roadsides, at forest edges, and in cultivated and wild fields in lowland and slightly hilly areas.

This plant is loaded with vitamins A and E, as wellas minerals like iron, calcium, magnesium, and potassium. It boasts amino acids, lipids, ascorbic acid, retinol, thiamine, riboflavin, niacin, carotenoids, inulin, and organic compounds such as aesculin, aesculetin, cichoric acid, along with bitter agents like lactucin and lactucopicrin (intybin) and their derivatives.

Radíki has a bitter taste and serves as a tonic.

It supports digestion, increases urine output, gently stimulates bile secretion and bowel movements, reduces asthma symptoms, and lessens inflammation. Its seed extract is believed to protect the liver.

Additionally, it can be concocted in a digestive or tea.

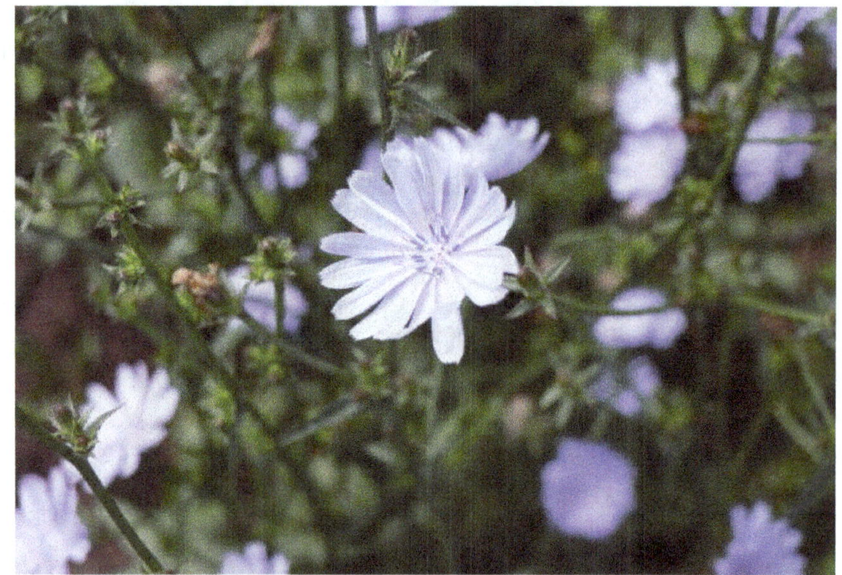

Herbal remedies for gallstones, gastroenteritis, nasal issues, wounds, and bruises include the flowers.

The leaves, tender buds, and roots are collected from **October to April** to be enjoyed fresh in salads or cooked with the shoots and roots, typically flavored with lemon and olive oil. They are often used in pies or prepared with lamb or goat meat as a fricassee.

Rapanída (Raphanus raphanistrum)

Rapanída—wild radish, white charlock, or jointed charlock—is a perennial plant marked by its dichotomously branched stem covered with stiff hairs, reaching up to 60 cm in height. The leaves have a lyre-like shape, with a pinnate structure, serrated oval side lobes, and a wider central lobe. Its flowers appear either white or pale yellow, often highlighted by violet veins.

It produces long, slender fruits that resemble a string of beads and tend to break apart easily when pressed. This plant flourishes in cultivated and unplowed fields, olive groves, waste areas, and along roadsides.

It is packed with vitamin E, polyunsaturated fats, particularly α-linolenic acid, and various phenolic compounds, chiefly kaempferol-3,7-O-di-rhamnoside.

Rapanída is valued for its antioxidant, antibacterial, caustic, tonic, and flavorful properties.

From **autumn through spring**, young shoots and tender leaves are harvested to be cooked and eaten as a salad, typically dressed with vinegar or lemon juice.

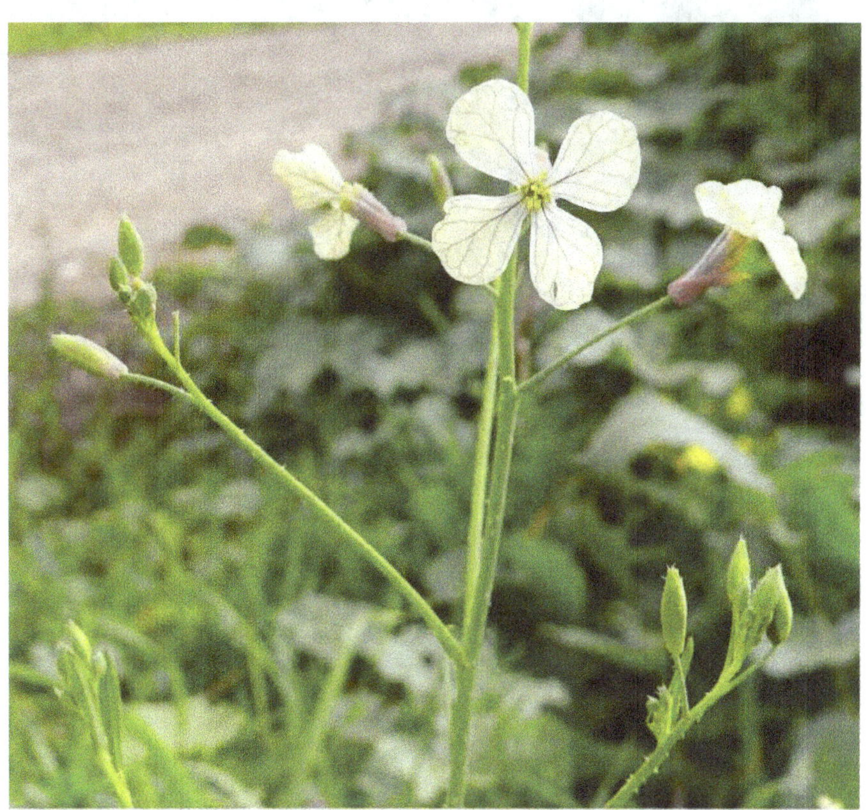

Photo by Math Knight

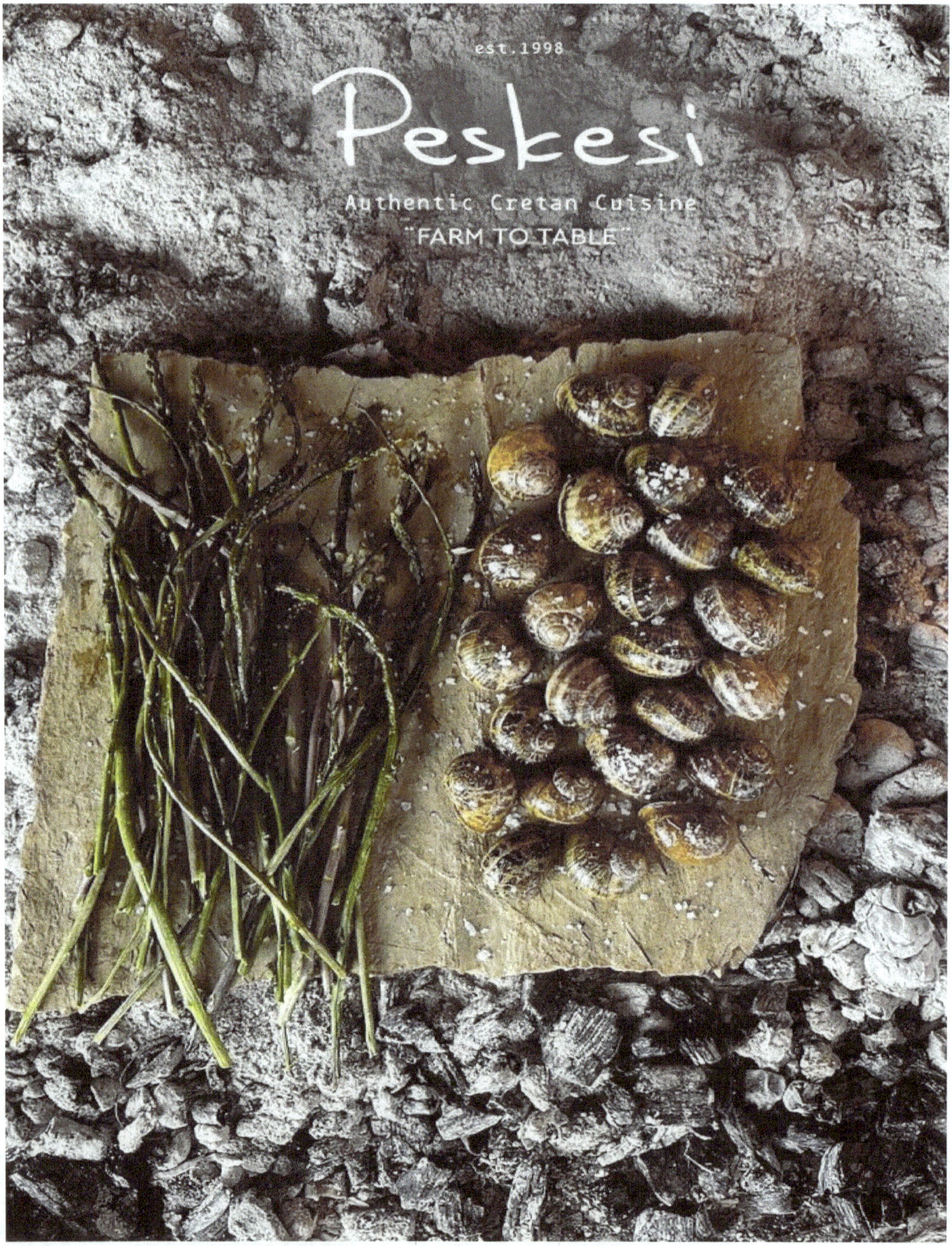

Peskesi in Heraklion incorporates seasonal horta in its menus.

Sparángi (Asparagus aphyllus)

Sparángi—Mediterranean asparagus, prickly asparagus, spiny asparagus—is a low-growing shrub with a dark green hue characterized by thorns in place of leaves. The plant is dioecious and has a substantial, succulent root system. The shoots emerge individually from latent subterranean buds without a central stem. Their color ranges from a pale white hue to various hues of green, and can even appear as a deep, nearly black green.

Its blooms are little and tubular and exhibit hues of white, greenish, or reddish at the lower extremities of the branches. Fruits are crimson tracks. Wild asparagus thrives in infertile environments, such as arid

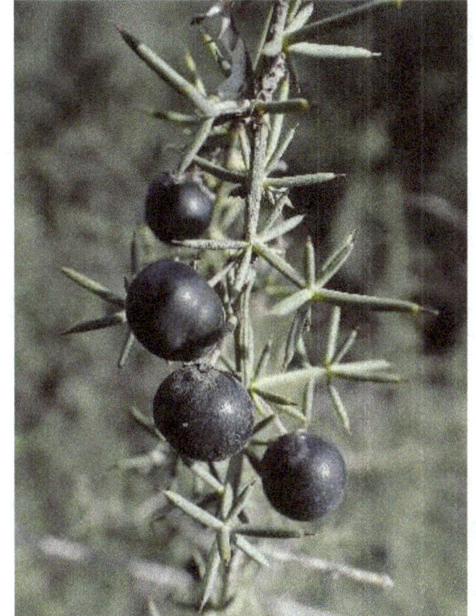

plains, olive orchards, slopes, clearings, and cultivated fields. It thrives on calcareous, acidic, or neutral soils with excellent drainage.

Sparángi is rich in vitamins A, B1, B2, C, E, carotene, magnesium, phosphorus, calcium, iron, sodium, potassium, zinc, folic acid, niacin, asparagine, arginine, tyrosine, resins, tannins, steroidal saponins, glycosides, and flavonoids.

Sparángi aids in controlling heartbeats, treats bladder and renal disorders, combats TB and bronchitis, and possesses antirheumatic and sedative properties.

The edible portion harvested **from March till May** consists of tender, immature shoots around 5-10 cm in length. It can be consumed in its raw state, typically accompanied by vinegar and salt, or incorporated into salads. Alternatively, it can be cooked with garlic and seasoned with vinegar or lemon. Asparagus is commonly consumed in the form of asparagus risotto, asparagus omelet, or asparagus soup.

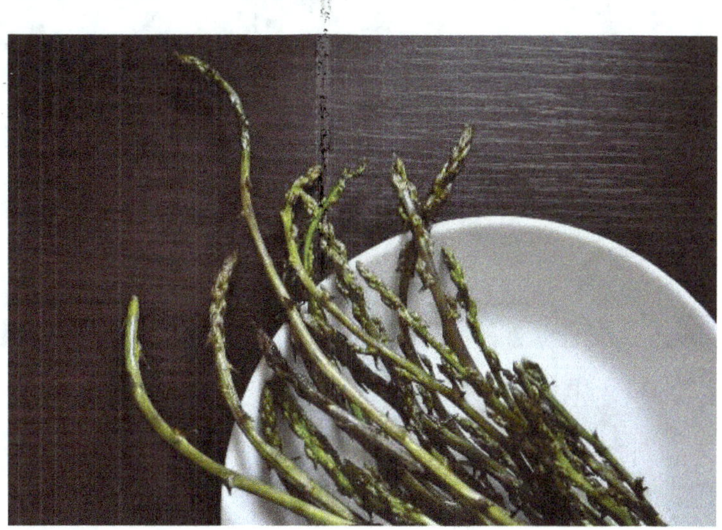

Stamnankáthi (Cichorium spinosum)

Stamnankáthi—spiny chicory—is a perennial shrub reaching 15-40 cm in height, notable for its intricate branching. Its shoots, smooth in texture, rise from the base with elongated grooves and feature spine-covered, blunt tips devoid of leaves.

Foliage appears on the lower parts of the shoots, attached by a short stalk. Leaves, measuring 3 to 15 cm in length, typically display a pinnate shape with toothed edges and a blunt deltoid terminal lobe. Lateral lobes often have dentate, continuous margins.

Spiny chicory blooms with solitary blue flowers from May to June, emerging from stem axils. Its fruit is a narrow achene with a truncated cross-shaped top. This plant thrives in coastal, mountainous, or plateau regions above 1000 meters in altitude and demands well-drained soil.

It withstands salt, cold, and snow but does not fare well in high spring and summer temperatures.

Nutritionally, Stamnankáthi is rich in antioxidants like vitamins A, C, E, β-carotene, phenols, and amino acids such as glutathione. It also contains linolenic acid and omega-3 fatty acids and is a good source of iron, zinc, potassium, and magnesium. It carries a low caloric load, offering about 6 calories per 28 grams.

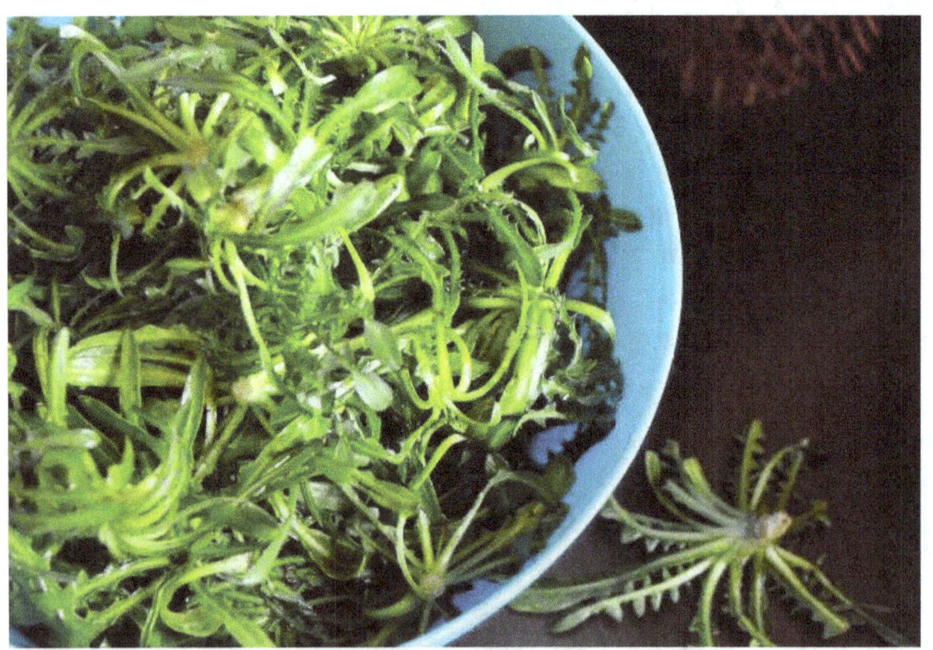

Stamnankáthi supports intestinal health, aids in slowing glucose absorption, binds cholesterol, and regulates weight.

It possesses antibacterial and antirheumatic properties and aids digestion and skincare enhancement.

The leaves and tender branches can be eaten raw or boiled with lemon and olive oil. They can also be cooked with goat or lamb meat in a lemony fricassee.

Starída (Hedypnois cretica)

Starída—Cretanweed or scaly hawkbit—is an annual herbaceous plant with variable hairiness, featuring flower stalks reaching heights of up to 40 centimeters. The leaves gather at the base, reminiscent of the common dandelion but with noticeable bristles. They can range in color from green to purplish and may grow up to 18 centimeters long.

The plant develops a single flower head or an arrangement of several heads atop its stalks. These heads are covered with rows of phyllaries, often very bristly, and are egg-shaped when unopened. Each flower head contains 8 to 30 yellow ray florets but no disc flowers. Blossoming occurs from April to May, creating a cluster of vibrant yellow flowers. Its fruit, an achene, is notable for its angular form and rough surface dotted with small ridges.

Starída flourishes in challenging, less fertile environments, such as rocky limestone areas, coastal fields, cultivated lands, vineyards, and the borders of fields in low and semi-mountainous regions. It also adapts to wet clay soils that retain moisture, growing up to altitudes of 400 meters. Chemically, the plant is composed of sesquiterpene lactones and isoetin, a flavone, which are considered essential for human consumption.

Between **February and April**, Starída is deemed both delicious and highly palatable. Its leaves and tender shoots are gathered for consumption before flowering, whether eaten alone or with other vegetables. They are typically boiled, fried, or included in dishes such as pies or kalitsounias

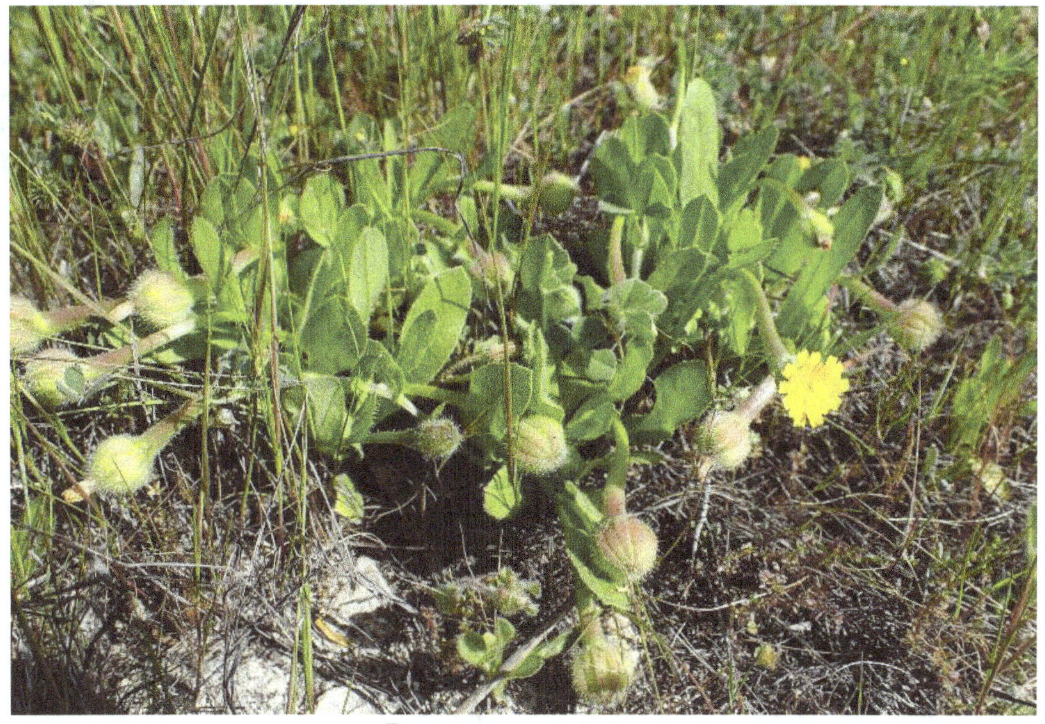

Photo by Krzysztof Ziarnek

Stafylínakas (Daucus carota)

Stafylínakas—wild carrot, European wild carrot, bird's nest, bishop's lace, and Queen Anne's lace—is a biennial plant that can grow up to 1 meter tall. Its green stem is upright, cylindrical, and grooved, often covered with hairs. The plant has numerous complex leaves alternating along the stem, featuring bi- or tri-pinnate leaflets that are linear or lanceolate. In the first year, it forms a circular rosette of leaves up to 45 cm wide.

During the second year, it blooms and subsequently dies. Its flowers, typically white and occasionally pink, organize in radial clusters with a deep purple central blossom. After flowering, the cluster closes inward, forming a nest-like structure. All parts of the plant have glands that release aromatic essential oils.

The wild carrot adapts to various habitats, including meadows, fields, and clearings in lowland and semi-mountainous areas. It prefers dry, temperate, and loamy soils.

Stafylínakas is rich in vitamins C, B1, B2, pro-vitamin A (carotene), sugars like glucose and sucrose, and pectin. It also provides minerals like calcium, potassium, iron, magnesium, phosphorus, and iodine, along with essential oils. It is beneficial for the kidneys and liver, helps relieve arthritis symptoms, improves vision, and assists in lowering blood pressure. However, **it should be avoided by individuals with diabetes.**

Before the blooming period, its tender shoots, leaves, and roots are collected for culinary use. The leaves and shoots can be boiled with vinegar and eaten alone or with other greens like broad beans or fresh peas. They are also used alongside other wild herbs, snails, or meat in dishes including vegetable pies, providing a unique aroma. The seeds are used to flavor soups and grilled seafood.

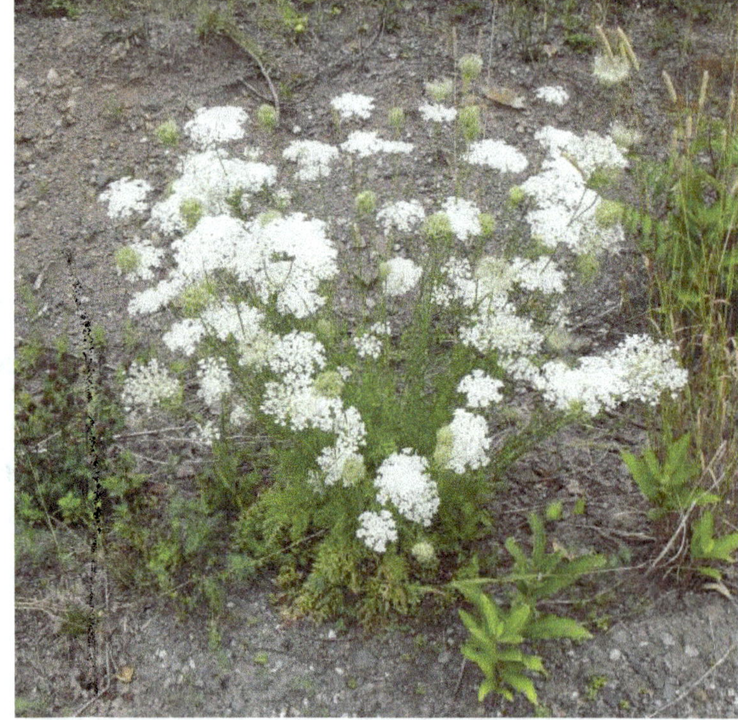

Photo by Gilles Ayotte

Striftoúli (Scorpiurus muricatus)

Striftoúli—caterpillar-plant or prickly scorpion's-tail—is a perennial herb. It features low-growing stems, often seen with fine hairs. Its leaves are simple, varying from spatula-like to lance-shaped, and taper at the base with 3 to 5 widely spaced veins and long stalks.

The prickly scorpion's-tail usually clusters 2 to 5 yellow flowers on long stems, typically blooming from March to May. Its fruit is a drupe, measuring 2 to 5 cm, notable for its spiral ridges and exterior spines. It prefers wet soils and thrives in cultivated fields, fallow lands, meadows, olive groves, and along roads.

Striftoúli is known for its pleasant taste. Its tender stems and leaves are harvested **from February to April**. People enjoy it hot in pies or as kalitsounia with other seasonal greens.

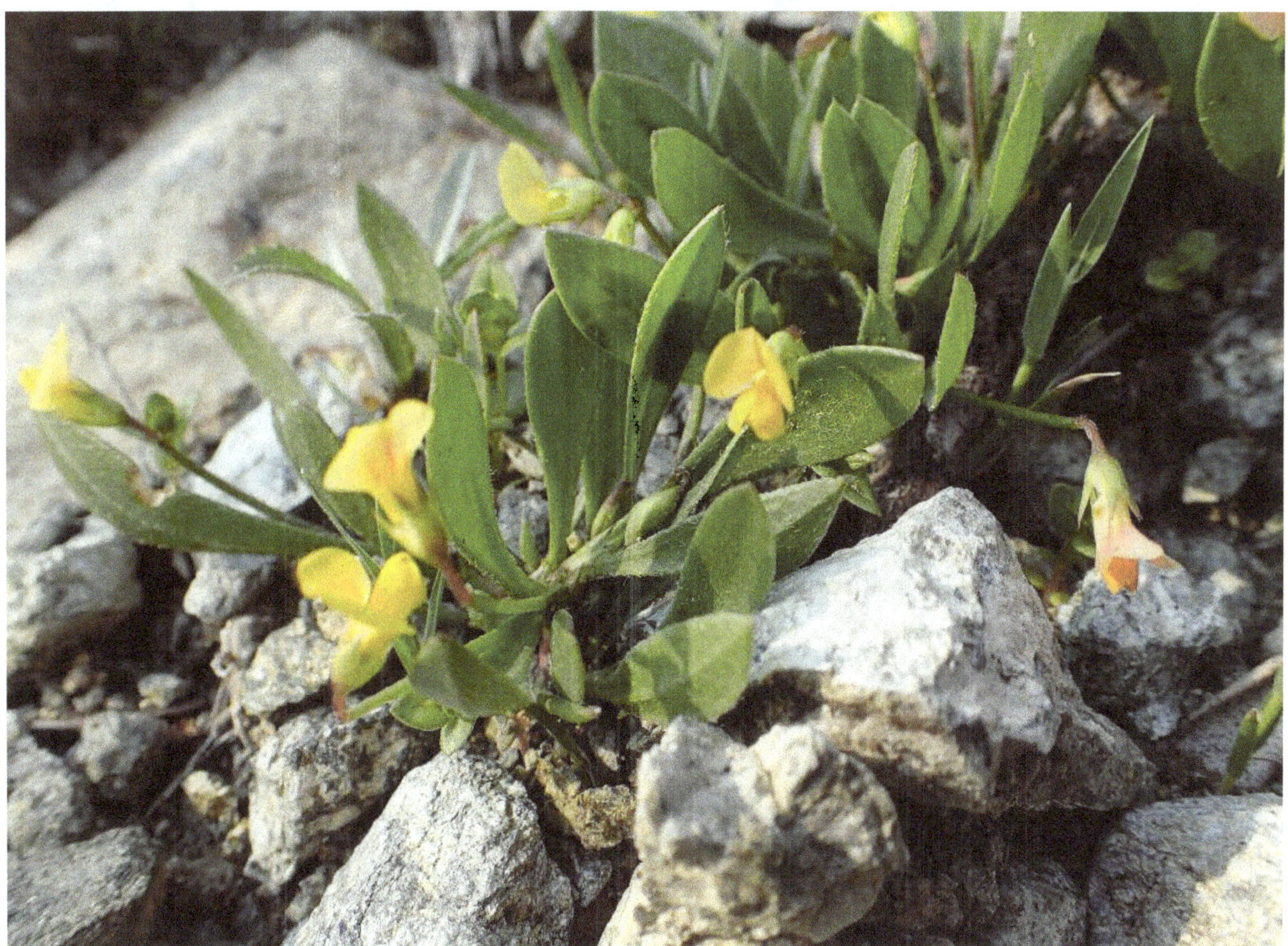

Photo by Krzysztof Ziarnek

Stroufoúli (Silene vulgaris)

Stroufoúli—bladder campion or maidenstears—is a perennial plant measuring up to 1 meter in height. It features multiple branches arising from a woody base, with leaves marked by a dark green hue and adopting an ovate, lanceolate form. These leaves have a soft texture; the lower ones are slender at their base. The flowers form in drooping clusters, mimicking tiny bubbles due to their unique spherical capsules.

Its calyx is smooth with a network of ribs and ends in triangular lobes. Each petal is large, elongated, and split into two lobes, displaying colors ranging from white to light purple. The plant's pale roots extend deeply, branching extensively beneath the ground, and it blooms **from March through August.**

Found in wild fields, by roadsides, and in rocky terrains at varying elevations, Stroufoúli thrives in less cultivated regions. It contains vital nutrients, including α-tocopherol, β-carotene, vitamins C and K, as well as essential minerals such as potassium, sodium, calcium, magnesium, and iron. Copper, manganese, zinc, and phosphorus are also part of its nutritional profile. However, it also contains saponins, so moderation is advised.

In culinary use, its leaves and young shoots are consumed fried or incorporated into kalitsounia, often mixed with other green vegetables. Stroufoúli can also form the base for a flavorful spongata (oven or pan omelet) or a side dish for cuttlefish and other fish.

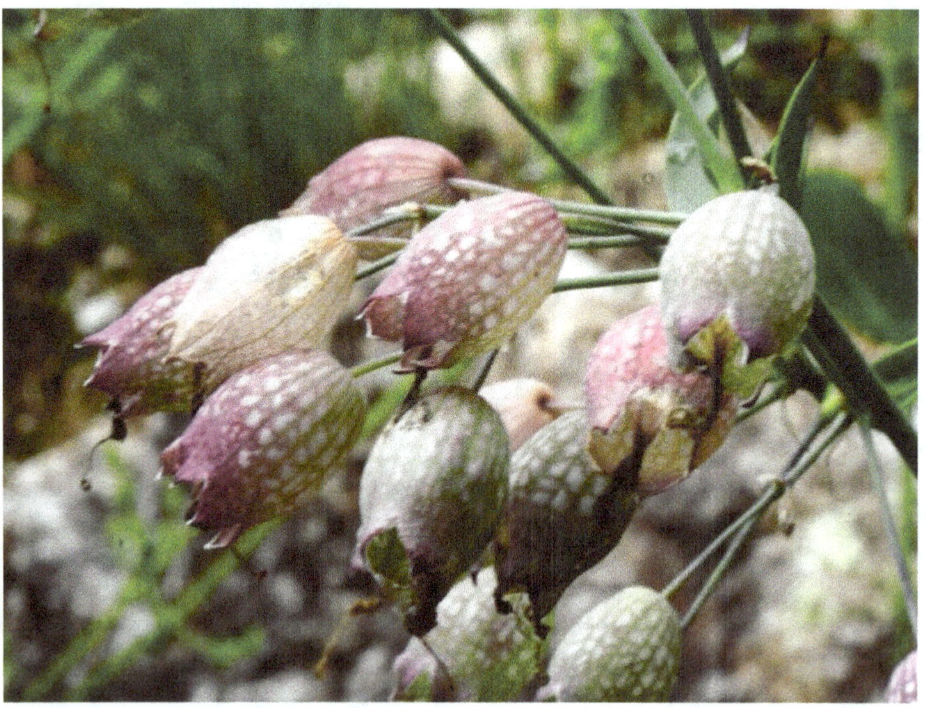

Photo by Enrico Blasutto

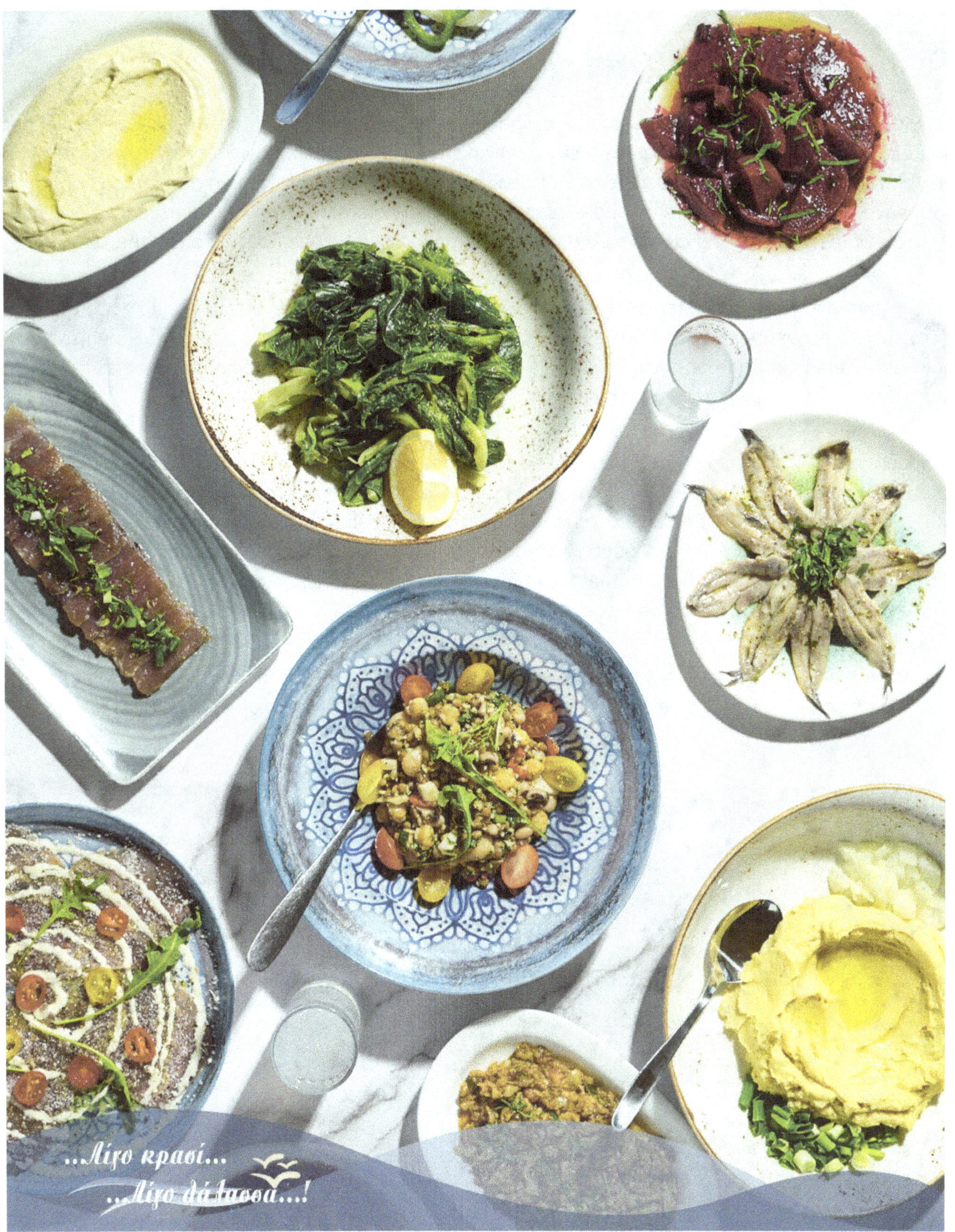

Horta takes center stage at Ligo Krasi Ligo Thalassa in Heraklion.

Stýfnos (Solanum nigrum)

Stýfnos—European black nightshade, black nightshade, or blackberry nightshade—is a perennial herb notable for its taproot and upright main stem, which stands sleek or slightly fuzzy. It grows to about 65 cm, branching out as it matures. Its leaves appear opposite one another, with an oval shape edged with soft waves. They have long stems and exhibit a rich green color. The plant's inflorescences emerge in the axils of leaves, featuring clusters of 3-5 white hermaphrodite flowers that bloom in the summer.

The oblong and juicy **fruits** start off green and **are toxic** due to solanine but turn black upon ripening from July to November. Stýfnos thrives in low-elevation environments such as embankments, slopes, cultivated fields, and gardens. It prefers well-drained soils but does not do well in shaded areas. The plant gains potency as the soil becomes more fertile and drier.

Nutrition-wise, Stýfnos is rich in proteins, carbohydrates, and several vitamins, including A, B1, B2, C, and E, along with niacin, carotenoids, omega-3 fatty acids, antioxidants, calcium, and phosphorus. The plant has various uses in traditional remedies, offering pain relief, reducing inflammation, promoting perspiration, increasing urine production, soothing skin, inducing relaxation, and dilating blood vessels. The plant demonstrates anti-inflammatory, immunomodulatory, and antiviral action to treat the SARS-CoV-2 infection and its post-complications.

The **leaves and young shoots are edible when boiled**; they are often added to salads and soups, sometimes combined with vegetables like beets or pumpkins or fried with other greens.

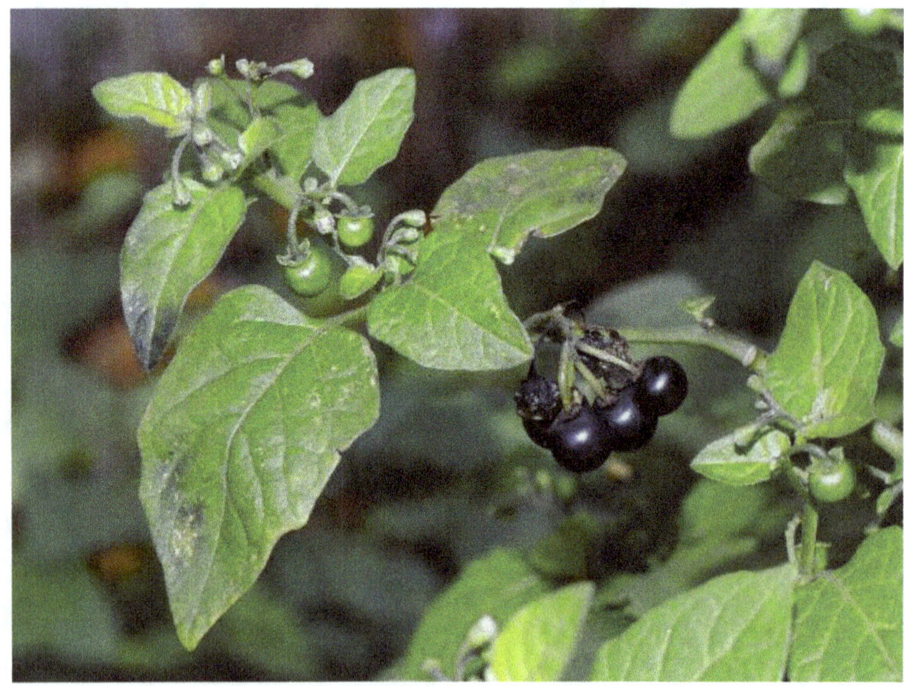

Tsichlántero (Stellaria cupaniana)

Tsichlántero—southern chickweed—is a perennial herbaceous plant. It can grow up to 50 cm in height. Its stem stays close to the ground and is cylindrical and green, covered in fine hairs, especially near the top where glandular hairs are present.

The plant's leaves grow in pairs, positioned in a cross pattern. These leaves are simple, lacking divisions or lobes, and are typically smooth. The lower leaves attach directly to the stem, but those at the top have very short stalks. The stem also has a purple tint and is smooth overall, with hair covering it.

The plant's flowers have a distinctive ray shape, organized in loose, wavy clusters. Each flower is made up of five white petals, divided deeply almost to their base. They bloom from January to April. The plant flowers within a delicate, elliptically shaped enclosure and prospers in cultivated fields, olive groves, meadows, and uncultivated and rocky terrains. It can be found along roadsides at altitudes between 50 and 1,200 meters.

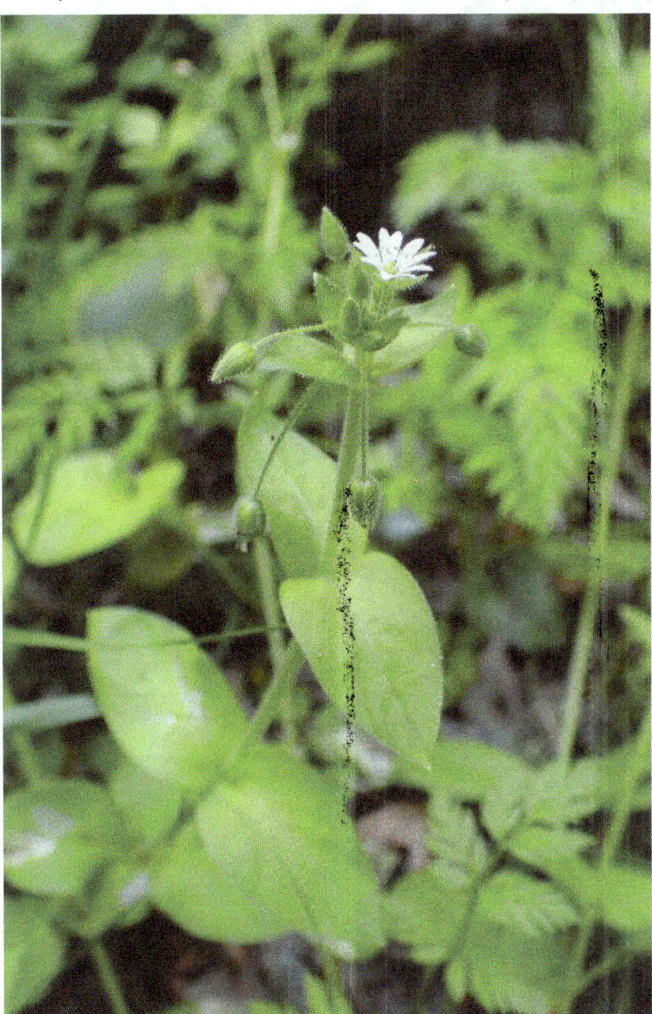

It contains saponin, vitamin C, rutin, aminobenzoic acid (PABA), γ-linolenic acid (GLA, omega-6 fat), niacin, riboflavin (B2), thiamin (B1), beta-carotene (A), magnesium, iron, calcium, potassium, zinc, phosphorus, salt, selenium, and silicon.

Dioscorides, a Greek physician from the 1st century AD, suggested its use with cornmeal for eye inflammation. He also recommended its juice for earaches. Nicholas Culpeper, an English botanist and physician in the 17th century, described chickweed as a soothing herb. He believed it could treat heat-induced pain, suggesting its juice for liver inflammation, facial redness, itchiness, and to relieve cramps, convulsions, palsy, and eye redness and swelling.

Traditionally, the young shoots of Tsichlántero have been eaten smoked and mixed with other leafy greens in a dish known as kalitsounia. Freshly added, it also enhances the flavor of salads. It is considered beneficial for promoting bowel movements, increasing urination, and alleviating rheumatic pain and weakness. Historical references to chickweed highlight its medicinal value.

Tsouknída (Urtica pilulifera)

Tsouknída—Roman nettle—is a perennial herbaceous plant known for its upright growth and basal branching. Its height ranges from 50 to 120 centimeters, with the plant's surface covered in rough hairs and showing a light green color. The leaves are heart-shaped, oval, or oblong, featuring a fluffy texture and jagged edges. They rest on a tall stem. The flowers are small and green, exhibiting dioecy, and appear in inflorescences during the spring. The plant's hairs contain histamine and formic acid, which trigger a burning sensation upon contact with the skin. This plan

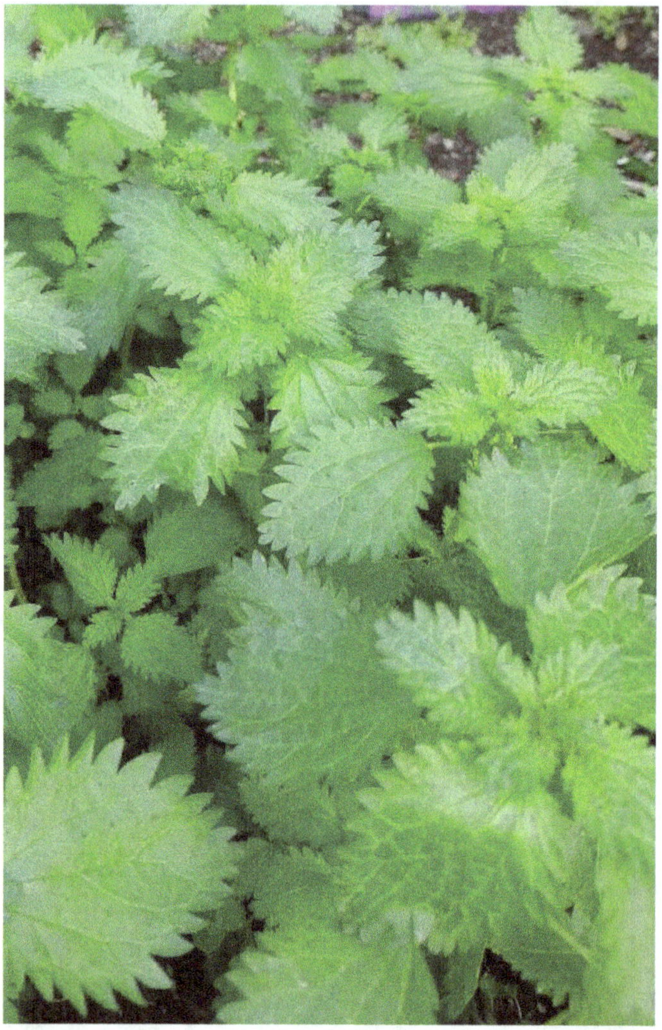

It flourishes in areas with either cultivated or uncultivated soil, especially in nitrogen-rich, lowland, and semi-mountainous regions. Tsouknída is an excellent source of vitamins A, B1, B2, B3, B5, C, K, and E. It also offers essential minerals such as calcium, iron, potassium, manganese, magnesium, phosphorus, selenium, and zinc. The plant is rich in phytochemicals, including lycopene, beta-carotene, caffeic acid, and betaine. Boiling or heating neutralizes the compounds found in its fine hairs.

Medicinally, Tsouknída is valued for its anti-inflammatory and antihistaminic properties, assisting in relieving rheumatic pain and soothing a cold-induced cough. It supports the management of inflammatory conditions of the prostate and urinary system, as well as allergic reactions.

Culinarily, Tsouknída's leaves and tender stems are often used alongside other leafy greens in salads, pies, and horticultural dishes. The leaves can be boiled and served with olive oil and lemon or included in sautés, vegetable pies, and dumplings. They also find their way into omelets and soups, providing a unique flavor profile that enriches these dishes.

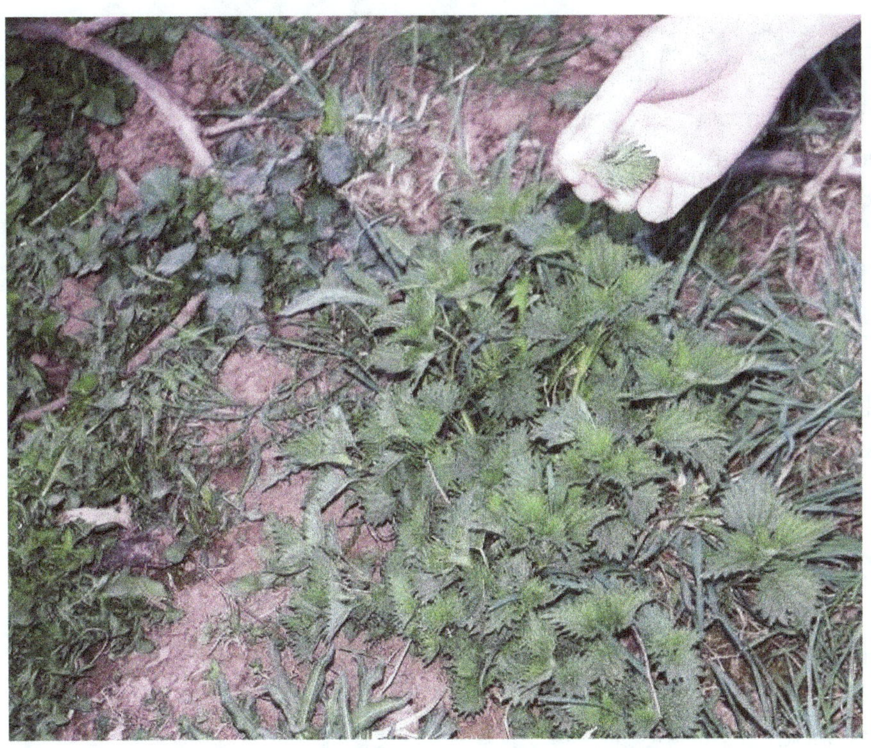

I like the bite of the nettle.
I eat weeds all the time:
the greener,
the wilder,
the better.
I'm probably a goat
grateful to live in Crete
where horta trumps grass
and I'll never go hungry
because
there's a pasture for every
season.

Tsóchos (Sonchus oleraceus)

Tsóchos—common sowthistle, sow thistle, smooth sow thistle, annual sow thistle, hare's colwort, hare's thistle, milky tassel, milk thistle, and soft thistle—is an annual herbaceous plant. It features a straight, striated stem that can reach up to 80 cm in height.

The stem branches minimally, is smooth with a reddish tone near the base in mature plants, and has a few reddish glandular hairs at the top. It also contains a latex-like sap. The leaves are generally spindle-shaped with serrated edges and pointed tips. They are smooth and clasp the stem at the base. The yellow flowers are small, sit in clusters at the stalks' summit, and appear from **February through June**.

This plant favors moist areas like cultivated or fallow fields in lowland and semi-mountainous regions, as well as roadsides, parks, and yards. It is harvested in late winter and spring. Tsóchos is packed with vitamins C and K, polyphenols, flavonoids, omega-3 fatty acids, and alpha-linolenic acid, which are vital for boosting the body's antioxidant abilities. It also contains minerals such as calcium, phosphorus, magnesium, iron, potassium, sodium, and zinc.

Tsóchos is known for its antioxidant and anti-inflammatory properties, diuretic effects, and ability to relieve muscle and joint pain.

Young plants, fresh leaves, and tender shoots are consumed. Their taste is slightly sweet. They are often enjoyed boiled in salads with other wild greens, dressed with lemon juice and olive oil or added to vegetable pies and sautéed mixed wild greens. You can brew young roots and use them as a coffee substitute.

Xynída (Oxalis pes-caprae)

Xynída—African wood-sorrel, Bermuda buttercup, Bermuda sorrel, buttercup oxalis, Cape sorrel, English weed, goat's-foot, sourgrass, soursob, or soursop—is a perennial plant that reproduces through small perennial bulbs formed by its taproots. The leaves arise near the plant's base, each with a long, smooth stem. Each leaf consists of three small, heart-shaped parts.

The flower stalk, devoid of leaves, is covered in fine hairs and holds yellow flowers. These flowers contain both male and female reproductive parts arranged in clusters called umbels. This plant thrives in diverse environments such as cultivated and uncultivated fields, gardens, olive groves, orchards, roadsides, and even rubbish dumps.

It contains potassium oxalate, oxalic acid, and vitamin C. Xynída possesses a range of properties: it is antiscorbutic, astringent, diuretic, emmenagogic, expectorant, antipyretic, irritating, and acts as a tonic that promotes the appetite and assists digestion..

In small amounts, Xynída adds a pleasant tartness to salads, sauces, soups, and vegetable pies. However, it is not recommended for people with kidney stones or rheumatism.

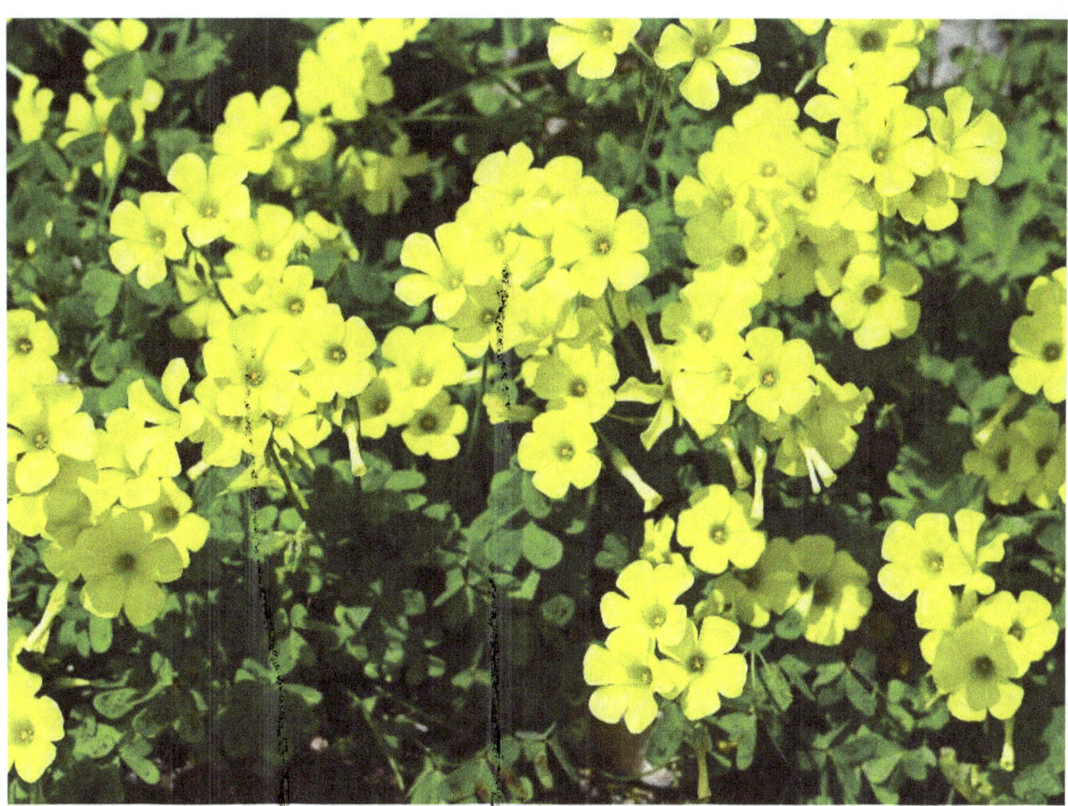

Photo by Krzysztof Ziarnek

Vlita (Amaranthus retroflexus)

Vlita, in English amaranth and scientifically known as Amaranthus retroflexus, is a versatile plant that grows either annually or perennially. It commonly reaches a height between 1 and 1.5 meters and features green, oval-shaped leaves. The plant's flowers, either iodine-red or green, appear in clusters or spikes.

Flowering occurs between June and September, while seeds are ready from August to October, with harvesting spanning from spring through fall. It flourishes in both uncultivated and cultivated fields. The wild form of amaranth is notably rich in nutrients like lysine, linoleic acid, other fatty acids, magnesium, starch, iron, and calcium, as well as vitamins A and O and tannins.

This plant is often prepared by boiling or frying, combined with various vegetables, and serves as an ingredient in vegetable pies with other leafy greens. Its nutritional profile makes it valuable for athletes, contributing to energy and endurance.

When made into a decoction, it can boost metabolism. Additionally, vlita benefits those with gluten sensitivity. The leaves have diuretic, tartaric, and antioxidant properties, adding to their health benefits.

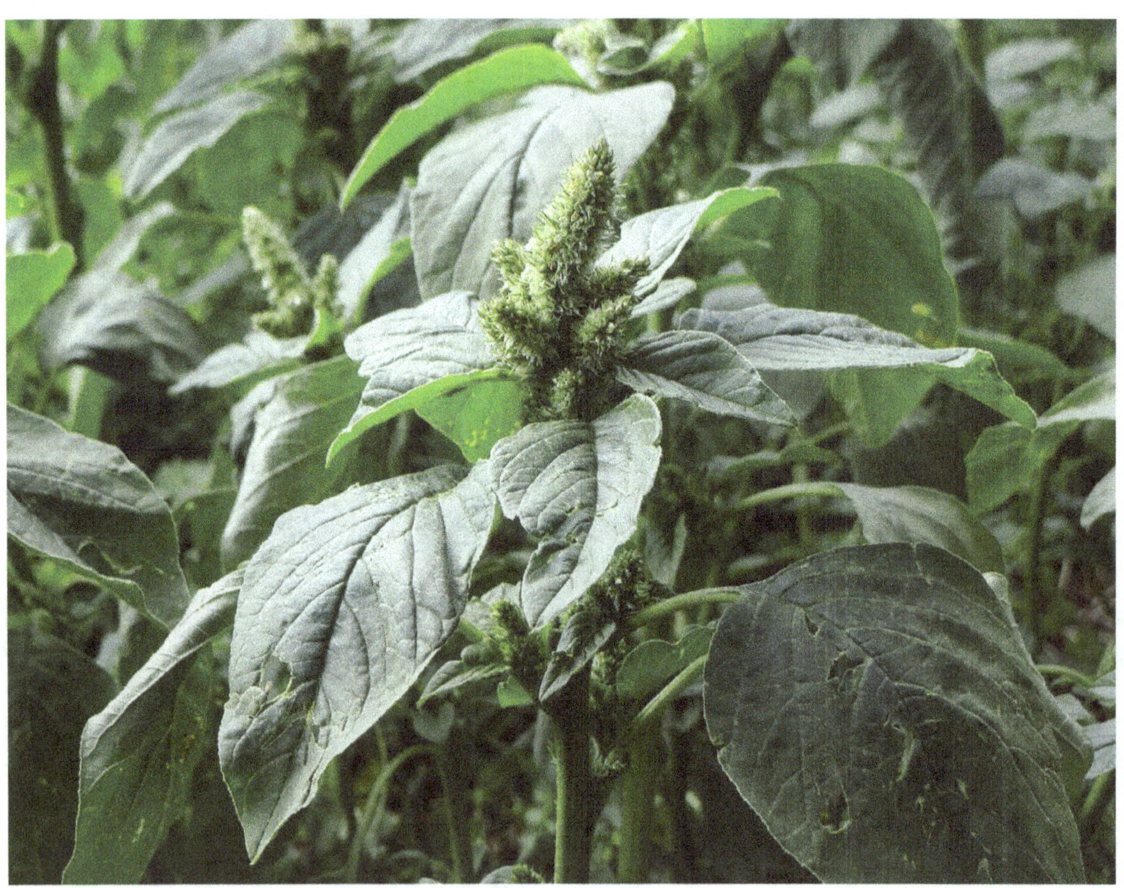

Horta with Tomatoes and Feta

Ingredients:

- 800 g amaranth greens (vlita)
- 50 ml extra virgin olive oil
- Two medium onions, diced
- Two garlic cloves, minced
- Four tomatoes, peeled and diced
- Fresh mint leaves to taste
- 350 g feta cheese
- Pepper to taste

Instructions:

- Blanch the greens in boiling water for 1 minute. Transfer them to cold water, then drain.
- Heat olive oil in a wide pot over medium-high heat. Sauté the chopped onions and garlic until fragrant. Add the diced tomatoes and cook for 5 minutes. Stir in the greens and simmer on low heat for about 20 minutes.
- Season with pepper. Since you will add feta, you don't need salt.

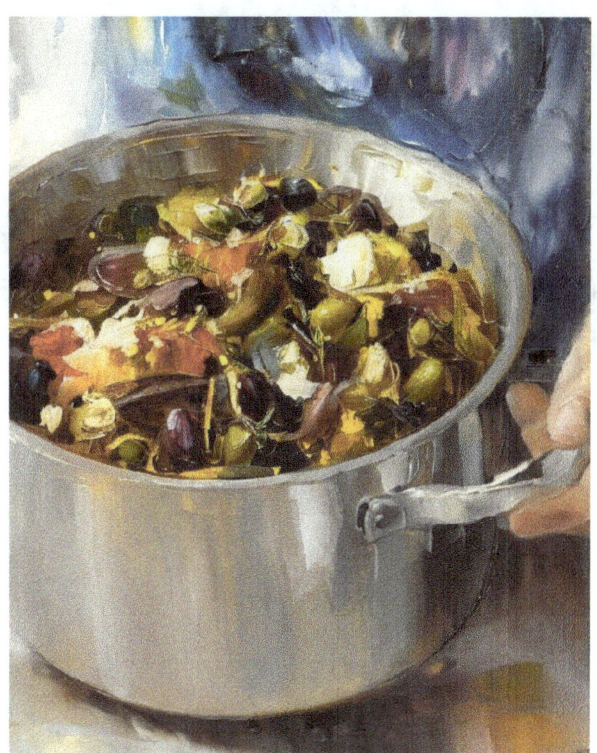

This dish blends amaranth greens, feta, and tomatoes to create a fresh, seasonal meal full of flavour.

- Remove the pot from heat once the greens are tender and the tomato sauce has thickened. Add the fresh mint and crumble the feta over the dish just before serving. Serve immediately.

Horta with Yardlong Beans and Potatoes

This salad can be enjoyed warm, at room temperature, or chilled. It pairs perfectly with grilled fish.

Ingredients:

For the Salad:

- 1 kg wild leafy greens (seasonal), washed
- ½ kg yardlong beans
- 3–4 large potatoes, peeled and cut into chunks
- 2 tbsp capers

For the Vinaigrette:

- One egg yolk
- 1 tbsp mustard
- Three garlic cloves, minced
- 1 tsp sugar
- 1 cup olive oil
- 40 ml vinegar
- Salt to taste

Instructions:

- **Cook the vegetables:** Boil the horta in a pot of salted water. Boil the yardlong beans and potatoes in separate pots until tender.
- **Assemble the salad:** Cut boiled potatoes into wedges or cubes. Combine all the boiled vegetables in a large bowl and add the capers.
- **Prepare the vinaigrette:** Blend the egg yolk, mustard, garlic, sugar, and salt in a blender. Gradually add the olive oil and vinegar, alternating between the two, until you achieve a smooth, runny sauce. Adjust seasoning if necessary.
- **Serve:** Drizzle the vinaigrette over the salad. Serve it warm or at room temperature.

Meat with Horta

This flavorful dish pairs perfectly with a chilled glass of Vidiano wine.

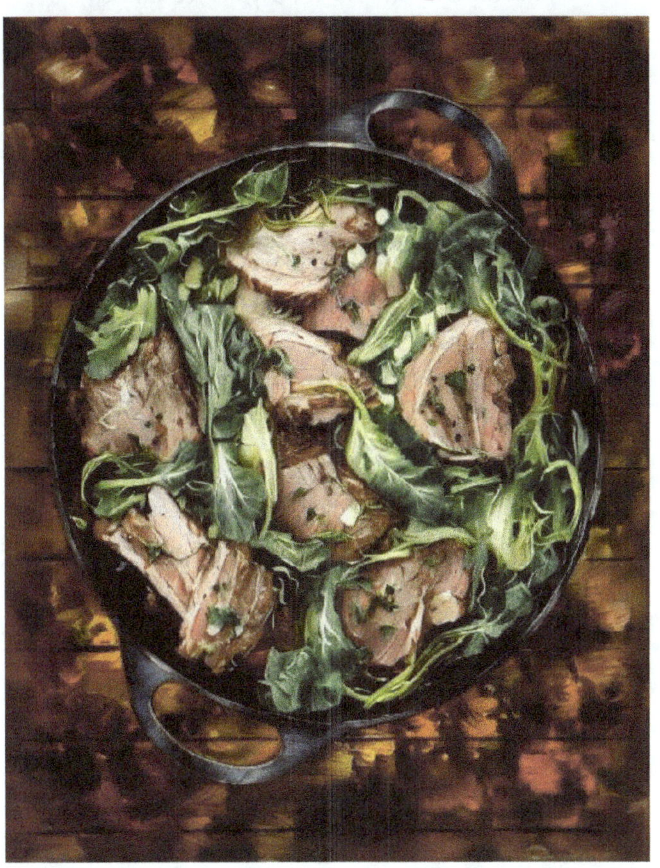

Ingredients:

- 1 kg meat of your choice (chevon, lamb, veal, pork, chicken), cut into medium pieces
- 1 kg seasonal horta, cleaned and thoroughly washed
- 1 tbsp Cretan herbs
- 200 ml extra virgin olive oil
- One glass of white wine (200 ml)
- Juice of 2 lemons
- Salt and pepper to taste

- Heat 150 ml olive oil in a pot until hot. Brown the meat pieces evenly on all sides.
- Pour in the white wine and cook for 2 minutes over medium heat until it evaporates.
- Lower the heat, add lemon juice, and season with salt.
- Cover the pot and let the meat simmer for 30 minutes. If the meat is too dry, ladle some vegetable broth or water.
- While the meat is cooking, wash and drain the greens.
- In another pot, heat 50 ml of olive oil.
- Add the greens, sprinkle with salt, and cook for 5-6 minutes until they wilt and release their juices.
- Transfer the cooked greens into the pot with the partially cooked meat.
- Continue cooking until the meat is tender.
- Sprinkle thyme and freshly ground pepper for a few minutes before removing from heat.

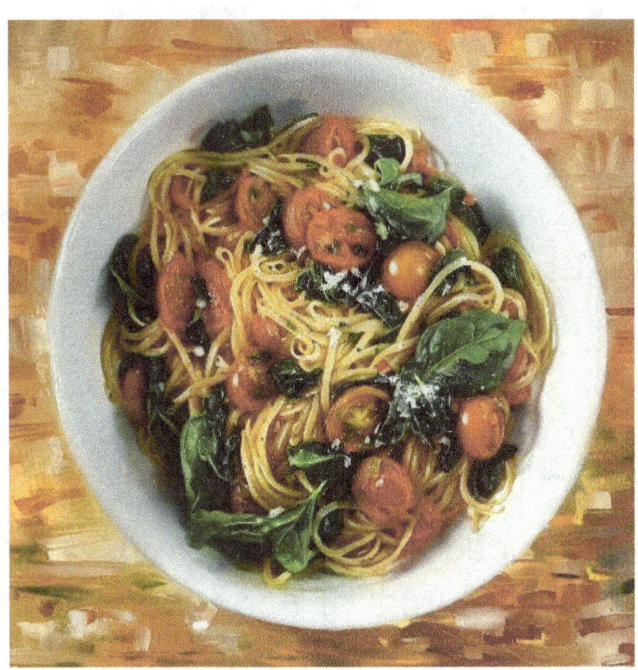

Pasta with Horta and Cherry Tomatoes

A light dish that pairs well with chilled dry white wines.

Ingredients:

- 250g dry pasta (half a package)
- 3 tbsp extra virgin olive oil
- 1 onion, finely chopped
- 1 garlic clove, minced
- 150 ml white wine
- 350g wild greens, roughly chopped
- 200g cherry tomatoes, halved
- 200g cheese, grated
- 2 tbsp mustard
- 150 ml cream
- Salt and pepper to taste

Instructions:

- Boil the pasta in a large pot of salted water until just under al dente, about 1-2 minutes less than the package directions. Drain, reserving 1 cup of the cooking water, and set aside.
- Heat the olive oil over medium heat in a wide, shallow pan. Sauté the onion for 3-4 minutes, stirring occasionally, until slightly golden. Add the garlic and cook for another 30 seconds. Pour in the white wine and allow it to simmer for about 1 minute, letting the alcohol evaporate.
- Add the wild greens and cherry tomatoes to the pan, mixing thoroughly. Cook for 4-5 minutes, letting the greens soften and reduce. Stir in the cheese, mustard, and cream. Season with salt and combine well. Reduce the heat to low and simmer for 5-10 minutes until the sauce thickens and the excess liquid has evaporated.
- Add the pasta, mix, and serve warm.

REFERENCES

- Hussain, Faiq & Ahamad, Javed & Osw, Peshawa. (2019). AMDHS ADVANCES IN MEDICAL, DENTAL AND HEALTH SCIENCES A Comprehensive Review on Pharmacognostical and Pharmacological Characters of Anchusa azurea. Advances in Medical, Dental and Health Sciences. 2. 10.5530/amdhs.2019.3.10.
- Sumengen Ozdenefe, M., Mercimek Takci, H. A., & Buyukkaya Kayis, F. (2022). Chemical composition and functional properties of Cynara cornigera lindley shoot system extract. Journal of Food Processing and Preservation, 46, e15867. https://doi.org/10.1111/jfpp.15867
- Almasri, Motasem & Abu -Shanab, Bassam & Hussen, Fatima & Qneibi, Mohammad & Eldin, Alaa & Yassin, Tariq & Khawaja, Momen. (2017). Phytochemical and Antibacterial Assessment of Rhagadiolus Stellatus Plant in Jerusalem Area - Palestine. Palestinian Medical and Pharmaceutical Journal (PMPJ). 2017; 2(1): 35-44. 2. 10.59049/2790-0231.1028.
- Zorzan M, Zucca P, Collazuol D, Peddio S, Rescigno A, Pezzani R. Sisymbrium officinale, the Plant of Singers: A Review of Its Properties and Uses. Planta Med. 2020 Mar;86(5):307-311. doi: 10.1055/a-1088-9928. Epub 2020 Feb 4. PMID: 32018307.
- Kapusta-Duch J, Kopeć A, Piatkowska E, Borczak B, Leszczyńska T. The beneficial effects of Brassica vegetables on human health. Rocz Panstw Zakl Hig. 2012;63(4):389-95. PMID: 23631258.
- Attiq A, Jalil J, Husain K. Annonaceae: Breaking the Wall of Inflammation. Front Pharmacol. 2017 Oct 20;8:752. doi: 10.3389/fphar.2017.00752. PMID: 29104539; PMCID: PMC5654839.

- Xie T, Wu Q, Lu H, Hu Z, Luo Y, Chu Z, Luo F. Functional Perspective of Leeks: Active Components, Health Benefits and Action Mechanisms. Foods. 2023 Aug 27;12(17):3225. doi: 10.3390/foods12173225. PMID: 37685158; PMCID: PMC10486880.
- Guijarro-Real C, Prohens J, Rodriguez-Burruezo A, Adalid-Martínez AM, López-Gresa MP, Fita A. Wild edible fool's watercress, a potential crop with high nutraceutical properties. PeerJ. 2019 Feb 1;7:e6296. doi: 10.7717/peerj.6296. PMID: 30723618; PMCID: PMC6361001.
- Güner ED. Oenanthe incrassans: An enigmatic species from Turkey and its comparison with Oenanthe pimpinelloides (Apiaceae). PhytoKeys. 2016 Apr 15;(62):101-11. doi: 10.3897/phytokeys.62.8106. PMID: 27212886; PMCID: PMC4856907.
- Baysal I, Ekizoglu M, Ertas A, Temiz B, Agalar HG, Yabanoglu-Ciftci S, Temel H, Ucar G, Turkmenoglu FP. Identification of Phenolic Compounds by LC-MS/MS and Evaluation of Bioactive Properties of Two Edible Halophytes: Limonium effusum and L. sinuatum. Molecules. 2021 Jul 1;26(13):4040. doi: 10.3390/molecules26134040. PMID: 34279385; PMCID: PMC8271801.
- Giglio F, Castiglione Morelli MA, Matera I, Sinisgalli C, Rossano R, Ostuni A. Muscari comosum L. Bulb Extracts Modulate Oxidative Stress and Redox Signaling in HepG2 Cells. Molecules. 2021 Jan 14;26(2):416. doi: 10.3390/molecules26020416. PMID: 33466890; PMCID: PMC7830645.
- Koyuncu I, Gönel A, Akdağ A, Yilmaz MA. Identification of phenolic compounds, antioxidant activity and anti-cancer effects of the extract obtained from the shoots of Ornithogalum narbonense L. Cell Mol Biol (Noisy-le-grand). 2018 Jan 31;64(1):75-83. doi: 10.14715/cmb/2018.64.1.14. PMID: 29412798.

- Berdja S, Boudarene L, Smail L, Neggazi S, Boumaza S, Sahraoui A, Haffaf EM, Kacimi G, Aouichat Bouguerra S. Scolymus hispanicus (Golden Thistle) Ameliorates Hepatic Steatosis and Metabolic Syndrome by Reducing Lipid Accumulation, Oxidative Stress, and Inflammation in Rats under Hyperfatty Diet. Evid Based Complement Alternat Med. 2021 Jul 10;2021:5588382. doi: 10.1155/2021/5588382. PMID: 34335826; PMCID: PMC8289590.
- Wahab A, Jan SA, Rauf A, Rehman ZU, Khan Z, Ahmed A, Syed F, Safi SZ, Khan H, Imran M. Phytochemical composition, biological potential and enzyme inhibition activity of Scandix pecten-veneris L. J Zhejiang Univ Sci B. 2018 Feb.;19(2):120-129. doi: 10.1631/jzus.B1600443. PMID: 29405040; PMCID: PMC5833326.
- El-Newary SA, Abd Elkarim AS, Abdelwahed NAM, Omer EA, Elgamal AM, ELsayed WM. Chenopodium murale Juice Shows Anti-Fungal Efficacy in Experimental Oral Candidiasis in Immunosuppressed Rats in Relation to Its Chemical Profile. Molecules. 2023 May 24;28(11):4304. doi: 10.3390/molecules28114304. PMID: 37298777; PMCID: PMC10254659.
- Karkanis A, Asprogeraka AC, Paouris E, Ntanasi T, Karavidas I, Rumbos CI, Athanassiou CG, Ntatsi G. Yellow mealworm frass: A promising organic fertilizer for common sowthistle (Sonchus oleraceus L.) and bristly oxtongue (Helminthotheca echioides (L.) Holub) cultivation. Heliyon. 2024 Aug 2;10(15):e35508. doi: 10.1016/j.heliyon.2024.e35508. PMID: 39170546; PMCID: PMC11336730.
- Oueslati S, Serairi Beji R, Zar Kalai F, Soufiani M, Zorrig W, Aissam S, Msaada K, El Modafar C. Antioxidant potentialities and gastroprotective effect of Reichardia picroides extracts on Ethanol/HCl induced gastric ulcer rats. Int J Environ Health Res. 2024 Feb;34(2):1088-1099. doi: 10.1080/09603123.2023.2198760. Epub 2023 Apr 4. PMID: 37015007.

- Saber FR, Elosaily AH, Mahrous EA, Pecio Ł, Pecio S, El-Amier YA, Korczak M, Piwowarski JP, Świątek Ł, Skalicka-Woźniak K. Detailed metabolite profiling and in vitro studies of Urospermum picroides as a potential functional food. Food Chem. 2023 Nov 30;427:136677. doi: 10.1016/j.foodchem.2023.136677. Epub 2023 Jun 23. PMID: 37390739.
- Zhou YX, Xin HL, Rahman K, Wang SJ, Peng C, Zhang H. Portulaca oleracea L.: a review of phytochemistry and pharmacological effects. Biomed Res Int. 2015;2015:925631. doi: 10.1155/2015/925631. Epub 2015 Jan 26. PMID: 25692148; PMCID: PMC4321094.
- Sun Y, Yang T, Wang C. Capparis spinosa L. as a potential source of nutrition and its health benefits in foods: A comprehensive review of its phytochemistry, bioactivities, safety, and application. Food Chem. 2023 May 30;409:135258. doi: 10.1016/j.foodchem.2022.135258. Epub 2022 Dec 20. PMID: 36587515.
- Noman A, Kanwal H, Khalid N, Sanaullah T, Tufail A, Masood A, Sabir SU, Aqeel M, He S. Perspective Research Progress in Cold Responses of Capsella bursa-pastoris. Front Plant Sci. 2017 Aug 14;8:1388. doi: 10.3389/fpls.2017.01388. PMID: 28855910; PMCID: PMC5557727.
- Maresca V, Vaglica A, Ilardi V, Bruno M, Basile A. Chemical composition and antioxidant activities of the essential oil of Tordylium apulum L. collected in Sicily. Nat Prod Res. 2024 Jun;38(12):2026-2030. doi: 10.1080/14786419.2023.2236765. Epub 2023 Jul 24. PMID: 37486088.
- Poonia A, Upadhayay A. Chenopodium album Linn: review of nutritive value and biological properties. J Food Sci Technol. 2015 Jul;52(7):3977-85. doi: 10.1007/s13197-014-1553-x. Epub 2015 Apr 7. PMID: 26139865; PMCID: PMC4486584.

- Pedreiro S, da Ressurreição S, Lopes M, Cruz MT, Batista T, Figueirinha A, Ramos F. Crepis vesicaria L. subsp. taraxacifolia Leaves: Nutritional Profile, Phenolic Composition and Biological Properties. Int J Environ Res Public Health. 2020 Dec 28;18(1):151. doi: 10.3390/ijerph18010151. PMID: 33379308; PMCID: PMC7796387.
- Kılınc H, Masullo M, Lauro G, D'Urso G, Alankus O, Bifulco G, Piacente S. Scabiosa atropurpurea: A rich source of iridoids with α-glucosidase inhibitory activity evaluated by in vitro and in silico studies. Phytochemistry. 2023 Jan;205:113471. doi: 10.1016/j.phytochem.2022.113471. Epub 2022 Oct 12. PMID: 36241054.
- Hmamou A, El-Assri EM, El Khomsi M, Kara M, Zuhair Alshawwa S, Al Kamaly O, El Oumari FE, Eloutassi N, Lahkimi A. Papaver rhoeas L. stem and flower extracts: Anti-struvite, anti-inflammatory, analgesic, and antidepressant activities. Saudi Pharm J. 2023 Aug;31(8):101686. doi: 10.1016/j.jsps.2023.06.019. Epub 2023 Jun 28. PMID: 37448842; PMCID: PMC10336831.
- Gnocchi D, Sabbà C, Mazzocca A. The Edible Plant Crithmum maritimum Shows Nutraceutical Properties by Targeting Energy Metabolism in Hepatic Cancer. Plant Foods Hum Nutr. 2022 Sep;77(3):481-483. doi: 10.1007/s11130-022-00986-z. Epub 2022 Jul 14. PMID: 35831770; PMCID: PMC9463332.
- Al-Qudah MA, Al-Zereini WA, Al-Jaber HI, Alhamzani AG, Bataineh TT, Abu-Orabi ST, Al-Mustafa AH. Isolation of a new flavonoid from Prasium majus L. with evaluation of its potential biological activities. Nat Prod Res. 2024 Jun 22:1-14. doi: 10.1080/14786419.2024.2364368. Epub ahead of print. PMID: 38907699.
- Jeong D, Irfan M, Lee DH, Hong SB, Oh JW, Rhee MH. Rumex acetosa modulates platelet function and inhibits thrombus formation in rats. BMC Complement Med Ther. 2020 Mar 23;20(1):98. doi: 10.1186/s12906-020-02889-5. PMID: 32204703; PMCID: PMC7092512.

- Tabanca N, Demirci B, Kirimer N, Baser KH, Bedir E, Khan IA, Wedge DE. Gas chromatographic-mass spectrometric analysis of essential oils from Pimpinella aurea, Pimpinella corymbosa, Pimpinella peregrina and Pimpinella puberula gathered from Eastern and Southern Turkey. J Chromatogr A. 2005 Dec 2;1097(1-2):192-8. doi: 10.1016/j.chroma.2005.10.047. Epub 2005 Nov 2. PMID: 16269150.
- Cano E, Musarella CM, Cano-Ortiz A, Fuentes JCP, Spampinato G, Gomes CJP. Morphometric analysis and bioclimatic distribution of Glebionis coronaria s.l. (Asteraceae) in the Mediterranean area. PhytoKeys. 2017 Jun 26;(81):103-126. doi: 10.3897/phytokeys.81.11995. PMID: 28785167; PMCID: PMC5523873.
- Mahboubi M. Foeniculum vulgare as Valuable Plant in Management of Women's Health. J Menopausal Med. 2019 Apr;25(1):1-14. doi: 10.6118/jmm.2019.25.1.1. Epub 2019 Apr 25. PMID: 31080784; PMCID: PMC6487283.
- Draginic N, Jakovljevic V, Andjic M, Jeremic J, Srejovic I, Rankovic M, Tomovic M, Nikolic Turnic T, Svistunov A, Bolevich S, Milosavljevic I. Melissa officinalis L. as a Nutritional Strategy for Cardioprotection. Front Physiol. 2021 Apr 22;12:661778. doi: 10.3389/fphys.2021.661778. PMID: 33967832; PMCID: PMC8100328.
- Mousavi SM, Hashemi SA, Behbudi G, Mazraedoost S, Omidifar N, Gholami A, Chiang WH, Babapoor A, Pynadathu Rumjit N. A Review on Health Benefits of Malva sylvestris L. Nutritional Compounds for Metabolites, Antioxidants, and Anti-Inflammatory, Anticancer, and Antimicrobial Applications. Evid Based Complement Alternat Med. 2021 Aug 14;2021:5548404. doi: 10.1155/2021/5548404. PMID: 34434245; PMCID: PMC8382527.

- Adom MB, Taher M, Mutalabisin MF, Amri MS, Abdul Kudos MB, Wan Sulaiman MWA, Sengupta P, Susanti D. Chemical constituents and medical benefits of Plantago major. Biomed Pharmacother. 2017 Dec;96:348-360. doi: 10.1016/j.biopha.2017.09.152. Epub 2017 Oct 10. PMID: 29028587.
- Saleem H, Zengin G, Ahmad I, Htar TT, Naidu R, Mahomoodally MF, Ahemad N. Therapeutic propensities, phytochemical composition, and toxicological evaluation of Anagallis arvensis (L.): A wild edible medicinal food plant. Food Res Int. 2020 Nov;137:109651. doi: 10.1016/j.foodres.2020.109651. Epub 2020 Sep 9. PMID: 33233230.
- Saleem H, Zengin G, Ahmad I, Htar TT, Naidu R, Mahomoodally MF, Ahemad N. Therapeutic propensities, phytochemical composition, and toxicological evaluation of Anagallis arvensis (L.): A wild edible medicinal food plant. Food Res Int. 2020 Nov;137:109651. doi: 10.1016/j.foodres.2020.109651. Epub 2020 Sep 9. PMID: 33233230.
- Dimitriadis, K. M., Karavergou, S., Tsiftsoglou, O. S., Karapatzak, E., Paschalidis, K., Hadjipavlou-Litina, D., Charalambous, D., Krigas, N., & Lazari, D. (2024). Nutritional Value, Major Chemical Compounds, and Biological Activities of Petromarula pinnata (Campanulaceae)—A Unique Nutraceutical Wild Edible Green of Crete (Greece). Horticulturae, 10(7), 689. https://doi.org/10.3390/horticulturae10070689
- Baycu G, Tolunay D, Ozden H, Csatari I, Karadag S, Agba T, Rognes SE. An Abandoned Copper Mining Site in Cyprus and Assessment of Metal Concentrations in Plants and Soil. Int J Phytoremediation. 2015;17(7):622-31. doi: 10.1080/15226514.2014.922929. PMID: 25976876.
- Zhang X, Pan Z, Wang Y, Liu P, Hu K. Taraxacum officinale-derived exosome-like nanovesicles modulate gut metabolites to prevent intermittent hypoxia-induced hypertension. Biomed Pharmacother. 2023 May;161:114572. doi: 10.1016/j.biopha.2023.114572. Epub 2023 Mar 22. PMID: 36963360.

- Ljoljić Bilić V, Gašić UM, Milojković-Opsenica D, Rimac H, Vuković Rodriguez J, Vlainić J, Brlek-Gorski D, Kosalec I. Antibacterial Fractions from Erodium cicutarium Exposed-Clinical Strains of Staphylococcus aureus in Focus. Antibiotics (Basel). 2022 Apr 6;11(4):492. doi: 10.3390/antibiotics11040492. PMID: 35453242; PMCID: PMC9027144.
- Birsa ML, Sarbu LG. Health Benefits of Key Constituents in Cichorium intybus L. Nutrients. 2023 Mar 8;15(6):1322. doi: 10.3390/nu15061322. PMID: 36986053; PMCID: PMC10058675.
- Iyda JH, Fernandes Â, Ferreira FD, Alves MJ, Pires TCSP, Barros L, Amaral JS, Ferreira ICFR. Chemical composition and bioactive properties of the wild edible plant Raphanus raphanistrum L. Food Res Int. 2019 Jul;121:714-722. doi: 10.1016/j.foodres.2018.12.046. Epub 2018 Dec 24. PMID: 31108800.
- Chileh Chelh T, Rincon-Cervera MA, Gomez-Mercado F, Lopez-Ruiz R, Gallon-Bedoya M, Ezzaitouni M, Guil-Guerrero JL. Wild Asparagus Shoots Constitute a Healthy Source of Bioactive Compounds. Molecules. 2023 Jul 31;28(15):5786. doi: 10.3390/molecules28155786. PMID: 37570757; PMCID: PMC10421306.
- Zeghichi S, Kallithraka S, Simopoulos AP. Nutritional composition of molokhia (Corchorus olitorius) and stamnagathi (Cichorium spinosum). World Rev Nutr Diet. 2003;91:1-21. doi: 10.1159/000069924. PMID: 12747085.
- Petropoulos SA, Fernandes Â, Tzortzakis N, Sokovic M, Ciric A, Barros L, Ferreira ICFR. Bioactive compounds content and antimicrobial activities of wild edible Asteraceae species of the Mediterranean flora under commercial cultivation conditions. Food Res Int. 2019 May;119:859-868. doi: 10.1016/j.foodres.2018.10.069. Epub 2018 Oct 26. PMID: 30884726.

- Badalamenti N, Modica A, Ilardi V, Bruno M, Maresca V, Zanfardino A, Di Napoli M, Castagliuolo G, Varcamonti M, Basile A. Daucus carota subsp. maximus (Desf.) Ball from Pantelleria, Sicily (Italy): isolation of essential oils and evaluation of their bioactivity. Nat Prod Res. 2022 Nov;36(22):5842-5847. doi: 10.1080/14786419.2021.2018588. Epub 2021 Dec 19. PMID: 34927490.
- Safronova VI, Piluzza G, Belimov AA, Bullitta S. Phenotypic and genotypic analysis of rhizobia isolated from pasture legumes native of Sardinia and Asinara Island. Antonie Van Leeuwenhoek. 2004 Feb;85(2):115-27. doi: 10.1023/B:ANTO.0000020278.58236.77. PMID: 15031655.
- Haroun-Díaz E, Torres Rojas I, Blanca-López N, Somoza Álvarez ML, Martín-Pedraza L, Ruano FJ, Vázquez de la Torre M, Cuesta-Herranz J, Bartolomé B, Blanca M, Canto G. Anaphylaxis due to Ingestion of Silene vulgaris. J Investig Allergol Clin Immunol. 2022 Apr 19;32(2):150-152. doi: 10.18176/jiaci.0715. Epub 2021 Jun 4. PMID: 34085937.
- Sharma D, Joshi M, Apparsundaram S, Goyal RK, Patel B, Dhobi M. Solanum nigrum L. in COVID-19 and post-COVID complications: a propitious candidate. Mol Cell Biochem. 2023 Oct;478(10):2221-2240. doi: 10.1007/s11010-022-04654-3. Epub 2023 Jan 23. PMID: 36689040; PMCID: PMC9868520.
- cabicompendium.51635, CABI Compendium, doi:10.1079/cabicompendium.51635, CABI International, Stellaria media (common chickweed), (2022)
- Bhusal KK, Magar SK, Thapa R, Lamsal A, Bhandari S, Maharjan R, Shrestha S, Shrestha J. Nutritional and pharmacological importance of stinging nettle (Urtica dioica L.): A review. Heliyon. 2022 Jun 22;8(6):e09717. doi: 10.1016/j.heliyon.2022.e09717. PMID: 35800714; PMCID: PMC9253158.

- Li Q, Dong DD, Huang QP, Li J, Du YY, Li B, Li HQ, Huyan T. The anti-inflammatory effect of Sonchus oleraceus aqueous extract on lipopolysaccharide stimulated RAW 264.7 cells and mice. Pharm Biol. 2017 Dec;55(1):799-809. doi: 10.1080/13880209.2017.1280514. PMID: 28112016; PMCID: PMC6130567.
- Clemente-Villalba J, Burló F, Hernández F, Carbonell-Barrachina ÁA. Potential Interest of Oxalis pes-caprae L., a Wild Edible Plant, for the Food and Pharmaceutical Industries. Foods. 2024 Mar 12;13(6):858. doi: 10.3390/foods13060858. PMID: 38540848; PMCID: PMC10969124.
- Baraniak J, Kania-Dobrowolska M. The Dual Nature of Amaranth-Functional Food and Potential Medicine. Foods. 2022 Feb 21;11(4):618. doi: 10.3390/foods11040618. PMID: 35206094; PMCID: PMC8871380.